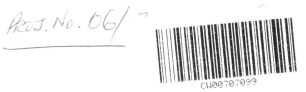

CHRISTOPHER'S STORY

THE CHILD WITHIN THE MAN

Published by
Chipmunkapublishing
PO Box 6872
Brentwood
Essex CM13 1ZT
United Kingdom

First published 2007

Copyright © 2007

http://www.chipmunkapublishing.com

INTRODUCTION

The word *autism* typically conjures up images of characters such as the one portrayed by Dustin Hoffman in the acclaimed film *The Rain Man.* Individuals with special gifts or talents are also the accepted norm when considering this fascinating condition. When people speak of autism they are typically referring to the syndrome Asperger's, where individuals are placed at the highest end of the autistic spectrum and are higher functioning and more able. Kanner's autism is poles apart from the above description and individuals have profound learning disabilities and other associated problems. Severe challenging behaviour is often present due to extensive communication difficulties and some individuals will also present with self-injurious behaviour. Sensory disturbances, such as noise and visual intolerance, will also often be present.

Most adults with autism were previously institutionalised due to their extensive care needs, specifically with regards to the issue of challenging behaviour and yet some families choose to remain together.

This book gives an insight into this fascinating condition and an introduction to our very special son who has been born ahead of his time into a world which is not quite ready for him.

In terms of age, an adult
but, as only parents can
when we look at you, we see
The Child Within the Man

CHAPTER ONE

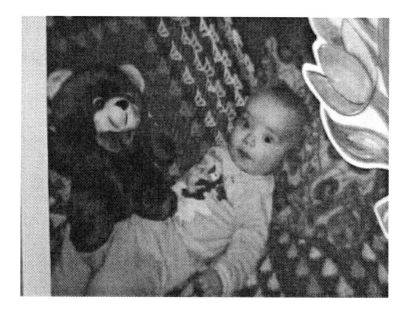

Christopher aged 5 months

 Our experience and knowledge of autism was virtually
non-existent until our youngest son became affected
and was later, diagnosed, with this life-changing
condition. Every person is an individual and every
person with autism is no exception. We were soon to
discover that the Autistic Spectrum is enormous and
that people with similar diagnosis to that of our son's
were typically very different.

        I suppose when Christopher eventually received
the diagnosis of autism, our immediate reaction was

one of relief. That might sound rather strange, but we were caring for a child who we knew to be very different from his siblings, but we had no explanation as to why this should be.

Christopher was the youngest of our three sons and he was born ten days before my due date on 1st June 1988. The pregnancy had been straight forward, although my haemoglobin level had been very low. It had also been low during my previous pregnancies, but it had been slightly more problematic this time and had resulted in my receiving iron injections at later anti-natal visits.

I was fortunate to have had short labours in the past, both having lasted around 5 hours and it was therefore envisaged that this one would at least be as expedient. I was advised to contact the hospital immediately when I showed any signs of labour and be prepared to make a hasty journey.

My contractions started at 10.30pm on 31st May 1988 and whilst Philip slept alongside of me in bed I lay awake wondering whether we would be welcoming a new son or daughter into the family. The hospital was just a few miles away and as there was initially quite a lapse between each spasm, I decided to wait until things progressed a bit further.

A couple of hours later I realised that this particular labour was progressing far slower than my first two had and so I remained in bed, clockwatching. There seemed little point in disturbing everyone until it was necessary. My sister had agreed to come to the house to take care of our sons so that Philip could be with me at the hospital and at around 5.00 am the following morning, I felt that things had progressed sufficiently to put our plans into action.

As expected, the roads were deserted and it took only a matter of minutes for us to arrive. I was taken into the maternity ward where routine tests were carried out. Labour had begun, but apparently it was going to be slow and I was given the opportunity to return home for a while.

The time passed by slowly and uncomfortably, but I ran myself a bath and did my best to relax given the circumstances. I had heard of labours lasting over 30 hours and grimaced at the thought. Having had no sleep the previous night I already felt exhausted and although I wasn't as yet in severe pain, it was too uncomfortable to settle or to sleep.

By mid evening we returned to the hospital once again where I was taken to the labour ward so that the baby and my progress could be monitored. We were assured that all was well - it was just going slower than had previously been anticipated and so the wait continued.

The rain fell steadily upon the window and trickled down in rivulets. It had become darker over the past hour and the only other sound which broke the silence, was the occasional scurrying of feet on the tiled floor of the hallway outside. Occasionally, the midwife returned to check how things were progressing, but for the most part Philip and I were left alone to chat and hold hands.

As the time of the birth approached Philip went in search of the midwife and at 10.40 pm Christopher finally decided to put in an appearance. The labour itself had been drawn out, but straight forward and we were relieved that no intervention had been necessary. As I looked down into the tiny reddened face I instantly fell in love. He was absolutely beautiful and a perfect completion to our family.

The following morning I lay Christopher on the bed to remove the little hospital gown he had been placed in and excitedly replaced it with one of the baby grows we had packed. Shortly after lunch, he arrived home to be welcomed into the family.

…..

Life was hectic and our young family was demanding, but we had wanted to have our children close in ages and we accepted that the early years were inevitably going to be the most difficult. Philip was working in Cardiff at the time and I remained at home, busily packing for what we hoped was to be our final house move. It was quite an exciting time with many things happening in close succession. First the new baby, then the house move and in just 3 months time, our eldest son Michael was due to start school.

The move itself went well and we soon settled into our new home. It was a much better environment for the children and being situated a short distance away from the main cul-de-sac, there were no roads immediately around the house. We believed that this would prove to be safer for the children when they were old enough to play outside in years to come.

Christopher was a contented baby and his interest in his family and environment was apparent. He enjoyed to watch his elder brothers playing *or* fighting together and loved nothing better than being cuddled and fussed over. He had a contagious giggle and an enchanting smile.

As the months passed by, we were concerned to note that there were occasions when Christopher would cough quite violently and vomit a thickened water-like substance. These episodes tended to last for several days at a time, during which, Christopher would lie around looking poorly and refusing to feed. It would take me upwards of an hour to spoon-feed him one bottle of milk and it was worrying to note the weight which he lost following these bouts.

We were surprised when the doctor finally diagnosed baby asthma as Christopher did not appear to have the difficulty in breathing which was apparent in members of our extended family. But we were relieved to learn that as he grew older, the episodes would become less frequent, until they eventually ceased altogether.

By the time 8 months had elapsed Christopher was finally sleeping through the night. He was always so full of energy and attempts to calm him before bedtime tended to fail dismally. We often felt that he was so reluctant to close his eyes because he was afraid of missing out on something interesting.

However, over the course of the following year, the baby we loved so much slowly began to change. His interest in walking around the furniture had diminished, the baby babbling had ceased, and the few words which he had learned were forgotten as he withdrew further and further into himself. He would, for the most part, sit or lie down and stare into space, oblivious of those around him. The skills which he had previously acquired were lost, along with his interest in favoured toys and activities.

It became increasingly difficult to settle him at night and the sleeping pattern which had been established for the past 10 months slowly deteriorated as Christopher began to wake for long periods, screaming for attention. We had been advised to leave him cry, as he would eventually fall asleep, but we soon discovered that by ignoring the crying and the resulting tantrums, Christopher was managing to weaken the structure of the entire cot and was placing himself in danger.

The cot was a large wooden one, and the damage that was being caused was not comparable with Christopher's size, but his strength was excessive, even by that time. He would grip the wooden slats of the cot, shake them violently and jump heavily onto the mattress, which loosened the screws. These were tightened on a regular basis and eventually replaced with larger substitutes, but when the wood began to split, we decided to purchase a bed. It seemed the safest option.

It was around this time that the health visitor became concerned by the lack of progress Christopher was making and a referral was made for a Consultant to visit us at home. We tried not to worry as the weeks passed by hoping that the problem would be a minor one, but we were admittedly a little scared of what we would learn.

The visit itself was quite harrowing when we were plagued by a barrage of questions and requests. Did Christopher have a specified number of words in his vocabulary? Could he dress himself? Feed himself? Stack blocks? Jump? Hop? Climb up and down the stairs? Time after time we responded in the negative and watched as the Consultant made notes on a form. The only person who seemed to be completely unaffected by the ordeal was Christopher as he walked around the lounge ignoring everyone's presence.

Finally, the consultant smiled at us and advised that Christopher was severely retarded. The meaning of the word was lost on me initially. I was relieved and ignorantly assumed the terminology to be less serious than that of mental-handicap. It was only when the Consultant stated that he would require specialist schooling and support for the rest of his life that the penny finally dropped.

We were completely and utterly devastated. Whatever we had been expecting to hear, it certainly hadn't been that. Christopher looked so 'normal', surely the Consultant had to be making some dreadful mistake? He was a beautiful little lad and we were being told that he would require specialist help throughout his life – it simply didn't make any sense.

Over time we slowly accepted that Christopher's difficulties were substantial and we grieved for the son we had lost. I think we experienced every emotion possible, from anger to fear and finally to an overwhelming urge to protect him from the world. It was like suffering from a bereavement and both my husband and I became depressed.

As Christopher became a large toddler the aggression which he had always on occasions displayed, became more apparent and people orientated. He would bite the back of his own wrist deeply, head-bang and slap walls and I seemed forever to be separating him from his elder brothers to prevent him from attacking them. But, it didn't matter how many times I picked him up and placed him elsewhere, he would repeatedly come back for more. Distractions didn't work and as Christopher no longer appeared to recognise any speech, I was unable to coax or negotiate with him. Our older sons frequently went to school with marks on their arms and face where Christopher had gouged them and as they were only 3 and 4 years older than their sibling, their understanding of his difficulties were limited.

Our family life became more and more strained as Christopher's behaviour impacted upon everything we did. Teacher-parent evenings, sports days or school plays were not an option, as Christopher would grab, kick and gouge anyone passing within arms-reach of his push-chair and he had begun to have screaming fits for no apparent reason. Shopping was also a nightmare as people either stared at this child throwing tantrums, or bent towards him in an effort to offer sympathy, unprepared for his sudden lashing out, despite our warnings. He looked just like any other child and was probably considered to be terribly spoilt. Outings became increasingly difficult and we felt constantly drained. It would have been easier to remain at home, but we persevered in spite of the glares and comments, but it was immensely upsetting and isolating nonetheless.

…But as difficult as Christopher's behaviour could be, there were also times when he could be an extremely loving child and when we were greeted with cuddles and kisses, it cancelled out all of the negative behaviours. He was a beautiful little lad who was unfortunate enough to be saddled with all of these difficulties.

By the time Christopher had reached 30 months of age he had undergone numerous blood tests, but the results had all come back negative and despite the increasing difficulties we were experiencing as a family, no cause for the extensive delay could be found. We were desperate and read any book or article which might give us an insight into what had happened to cause the problems. I recall wondering if he might have been suffering from glue-ear. Well, that would have explained his lack of speech and his inability to understand others - if he couldn't actually *hear* them, that is. But, although a hearing problem might have explained the delay with his speech, it wouldn't explain his lack of progress in all the other areas of his development, or his lack of awareness of danger.

Although Christopher had learned to walk by the time he had reached 18 months, he frequently stumbled or tripped. He could walk or run on flat surfaces – with supervision – but he always fell when attempting to negotiate gradients. Stairs and steps were also a great cause of worry as Christopher would happily walk off the top step without being conscious that there was a drop. He simply stared ahead, oblivious of the dangers. We were not too concerned with this initially, as Christopher was always carefully supervised when negotiating steps, but when no improvements were made, we finally accepted that the stair gates would have to remain in place for a little longer at least.

We adapted Christopher's environment to best suit his needs. Anything which could be broken was placed out of reach, along with objects which could be used as weapons. It also became necessary to lock doors to prevent him from absconding and injuring himself outside.

When we visited family it was always necessary to *shadow* him throughout the visit to prevent him from damaging peoples' belongings or hurting himself, but we felt that it was important for him to get to know his extended family and for them to get to know him, and so we persevered.

We hoped that as time elapsed Christopher would learn about danger and become slightly more independent, but it was difficult to forget what the Consultant had said or the implications it would have for his and our future.

CHAPTER TWO

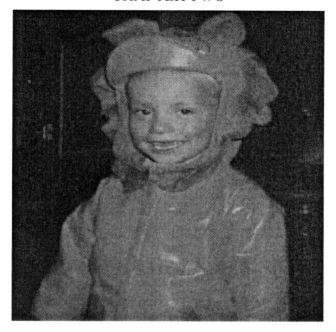

Christopher aged 3 years

In September 1991 Christopher had reached the appropriate age for attending nursery, but it was during this time that we suddenly discovered that his complex needs would seriously impact upon the services which were readily available to other children. Nursery placements in the area were typically well sought after but as children with speech, social and learning difficulties are generally given priority, we were not concerned about securing a placement. The application form had been completed and returned and we were just waiting to discover if he would receive morning or afternoon provision.

An educational psychologist had asked to visit us at home but as other professionals often made the same request, we did not suspect that the visit was in any way connected to the nursery placement. However, it was not long into the visit before we were being informed that Christopher could not attend nursery as the Department had no resources available to fund the 1-1 assistant which he needed. The psychologist went on to stress that given the extent of Christopher's learning delay and social development, it might be more beneficial for us to delay nursery until the following year in any event. At which time the financial situation could prove to be different and he could simply start a year later than usual.

The situation was not ideal but we appeared to have no choice other than to accept it. After all, if there was no money available to fund an assistant, it would not be a safe environment for Christopher *or* the other children. It was disappointing to have spent the past few months preparing for this milestone, only for it to be delayed in this way and so we considered what other opportunities were available in the meantime.

We were informed of a playgroup which was only a few miles from where we lived and decided to introduce Christopher. It was a friendly group and the children who attended were all pre-school age, with a variety of disabilities. The room which had been allocated was used as a typical play group on other days of the week, but on Wednesday mornings it was used by families such as ours. The room itself was enormous and whilst a small section housed a few tables and chairs from which the parents could watch the children playing, the remainder was filled with a lovely selection of toys, activities, bikes and other sit-and-ride vehicles.

The other children were able to amuse themselves and many played together, but Christopher typically roamed around, throwing various objects and toys as he inevitably did in all environments. Attempts to lash out at the other children meant that it was necessary for Philip and me to take it in turns to follow him throughout each session. But whilst one of us kept a close watch on what he was doing, it provided the other parent with the opportunity to sit and chat with the mums and dads, if only for a brief time. Having realised that we lived only a couple of roads away from one of the mothers and her little boy, arrangements were made for us to travel together and we soon became used to the Wednesday morning routine and being part of the group, which was a good source of support and advice in the early years.

Soon we were preparing for Christopher to begin nursery again. It was an exciting time, but also a worrying one. He still had no communication ability and his tendency to attack without provocation remained. He could harm others but he was also very vulnerable. We were anxious to say the least.

The summer holidays were fast approaching, but although details of the type of provision which was to be offered had not as yet arrived, we were not too concerned at first. But as the weeks continued to pass and we had still not received any communication from the nursery, we decided to make contact ourselves, where we were informed that there was no placement.

Our confusion was closely followed by despair when, having contacted the Education Department, it was confirmed that Christopher did not have a nursery placement. In our ignorance, we had assumed that *as* the Education Department had requested that Christopher start nursery a year later, the Education Department would have therefore reserved a placement the following year. Apparently, the reality of the situation was that we had been expected to re-apply for a placement ourselves once again and wait to discover if there were sufficient resources available for Christopher to attend. The misunderstanding and evident disappointment made little difference to the scenario in any event. If there had been sufficient funding for him to receive support at nursery this year, without our re-applying for a placement it was no longer relevant, as all of the places had now been taken.

With Christopher being school age and no provision having been organised, we were now greatly concerned. He could continue to attend the special needs playgroup, but that was only for 2 hours each week and it did not provide the specialist input and access to speech and language therapies which he desperately needed.

The Education Department requested that we view a special needs school instead and a date was scheduled for us to do so, but in truth, we had dismissed this particular school before we had even seen it. Two mums at the special needs playgroup had children there and we were horrified to learn that they had been returned home in soiled and wet clothing. Both mums had obviously been very upset by the condition their children had arrived home in and one of them was searching for an alternative school.

A young nursery nurse who we also became friendly with had completed training at the school and told us that a little girl had stood during song-time and had been roughly pulled back down to her seat. We reluctantly agreed to visit the school, but we still had great concerns about our son becoming a pupil there.

Nevertheless, we arrived as arranged and did our best to be as optimistic as we could. The school catered for children with moderate to severe disabilities and despite our misgivings, the head-teacher seemed approachable and pleasant. The classroom which Christopher would be joining if he became a pupil at the school was a little smaller than we had expected and did not afford much space for the youngest pupils or those who remained in wheelchairs, but here again, the staff seemed pleasant.

However, we were concerned when the issue surrounding Christopher's behavioural difficulties was discussed, to be informed that he would remain in the classroom throughout the day. This included lunch time, where it was planned that a meal could be brought into the room so that he could eat at one of the tables to avoid having to use the canteen with the other children.

Considering the class size and lack of space the room had to offer we did not feel that this solution was appropriate and if Christopher was not given the opportunity to mix and socialise with other children at such times, we were not confident that these skills could be improved upon. We were disappointed as the tour continued and had decided that the school was not for our son.

The Education Department was immediately informed of our decision but within weeks of contacting them we were stunned to receive a letter supplying details of a start date and school times for Christopher. The letter also contained details regarding the school bus and advised the time it would arrive to collect him on the date specified. We contacted the Education Department to again stress that Christopher would not be joining the school and were even more surprised to receive a Statement of Educational Needs shortly afterwards. The Statement gave the school name as being the most appropriate to meet Christopher's needs, and contained only 5 sheets of paper. As we studied the list of professionals who had contributed to its existence, we realised that none of them had actually seen our son. Little wonder that instead of providing details of his abilities in the relevant sections on the Statement, each professional had written *unable to comment*.

We once again contacted the Education Department to state that Christopher would not be joining the school as arranged, without our knowledge or consent, but would be remaining at home if no other provision could be located. Following this final refusal, the Department found a placement at a local playgroup.

The group met daily in the community hall opposite the cul-de-sac where we lived and Christopher was offered 2-hourly sessions, with a support worker, which took place on Mondays and Wednesdays. He settled in well over time, considering that the people and surroundings were unfamiliar and he became particularly fond of one of the support workers. She worked hard and always encouraged him to experiment with different materials, such as using paint and crayons on paper, using the hand-over-hand technique.

Philip and I used the time when Christopher was at playgroup to search for other schools in the area and family and friends were making enquiries on our behalf too. One of the nicest of the schools we visited was situated near Newport, but as it only catered for children with mild to moderate learning difficulties our search continued.

We were still in regular contact with the Education Department as Christopher had been due to commence his schooling in September of the previous year and just as we had given up hope of locating an appropriate school, we were told of one situated in Ebbw Vale. Philip contacted the school and made an appointment for us to view it, but having already viewed several which were unable to cater for children with more complex needs, we were not optimistic of the outcome. Nevertheless, we arrived at the appointed time, whilst Christopher remained at the playgroup.

We sat through the compulsory discussion with the head-teacher and were then given the opportunity to look around the building and grounds. The school itself was remarkably spacious with good sized rooms and wide corridors for easy wheelchair and pupil access. It had a cheerful interior which was accomplished by a combination of good lighting and large windows and this made it less oppressive than some we had seen. The over all effect was impressive and despite our initial pessimism, as we went from classroom to classroom our enthusiasm couldn't help but grow. We realised that the school not only catered for children with more severe disabilities, but that the teachers were compassionate and most importantly, the pupils were happy.

It was lovely to note that the head-teacher knew the children by name throughout the school and to hear him discuss individual interests with them. It was also lovely to see them respond with smiles and evident fondness to the playful banter. We were ecstatic and at that point had decided that we could entrust Christopher to their care without any further reservations. A decision had finally been made, at least on our part.

From the school's perspective, the head-teacher wanted to meet with Christopher before deciding whether a placement could be offered to him. It was thought that a meeting at the playgroup a few days later would be a beneficial place for this to happen and this would give the class teacher an opportunity to observe her potential charge.

As the day arrived we waited at home nervously, but quietly optimistic of the outcome and in the afternoon the call we had been waiting for finally came. The school felt that they could '*do something with Christopher*' and were happy to be able to accept him as a pupil. We were thrilled and immediately wrote to the Education Department to inform them that we had located a suitable special needs school for our son. However, instead of receiving the expected letter with start date, when a response finally arrived it was to deny Christopher access to the school of our choice.

During the following weeks we remained in constant contact with the Education Department in an attempt to resolve the situation, but despite being advised that we had the right to choose an alternative school if it was deemed to be appropriate, the dispute continued. The excuses came fast and furious and ranged from our chosen school being further away than the Department's offered school, to advising that if we refused to send our son to the local school then other parents might also wish to do so. This could then result in a possible closure due to falling pupil numbers.

I argued that if existing parents wished to remove their children from the school and new parents did not wish their children to attend the school, then surely this should be investigated? There was a placement available at the school of our choice and Christopher had been seen and accepted as a potential pupil there, I insisted that we would not reconsider. Unfortunately, neither would the Education Department, and so Christopher's access to the Ebbw Vale school was denied.

During the following weeks we contacted anyone that we thought might be able to offer assistance, from the Chief Executive of the Council through to our general practitioner, but all to no avail. No amount of letters and telephone calls made any difference to our plight and we were at a loss as to our next move. With little to lose we decided to ascertain the distances of both schools from our home, as although our preferred school was not in the catchment area, we were not convinced that it was any further away. In fact, as the school route incorporated a long mountain road which was without queues and traffic lights, it took us less time to arrive there than it had the catchment school.

Having harnessed Christopher into the back seat of the car we set the clock on zero and headed up the valleys. The view of the mountains never ceases to impress me and as we neared our destination it was easy to imagine that we were in the heart of Scotland, or some equally beautiful part of the country. Nevertheless, we concentrated on the task at hand and no sooner had we arrived in the school car park, then we noted the distance on the clock, turned the car around and drove home.

It was necessary to return to the cul-de-sac where we had originally started out from to begin the whole process again, but this time with the catchment area school as our destination. There were no mountains or scenic landscape to act as a backdrop on this occasion, just an accumulation of junctions and buildings, but the view was not an issue in the task, it was simply an observation.

On arrival at the school car park we again noted the distance we had covered and were delighted to discover that the Ebbw Vale School was actually a mile nearer to our home. When the absence of queues and traffic lights were also taken into account, the travelling time was reduced still further and armed with these facts we again contacted the Education Department. Unfortunately, our continued efforts were rendered useless as Christopher's access to the school continued to be denied.

As the weeks passed by people who lived in the area and heard of the difficulties we were encountering were very sympathetic and we suddenly realised that public opinion might sway the Department's decision. After all, the reasons we had been given were pretty lame ones and we had nothing left to lose. The local press office took an immediate interest in the difficulties we were experiencing and this resulted in an article being published about Christopher's plight. The support for our family grew still further. The article had raised awareness about the Educational Department's refusal to grant parents the right to choose a school for their disabled offspring. And following the positive response from the coverage, the journalist contacted the Department for comments.

Within a few days of the story being published we received the call we had been praying for - Christopher had finally been granted permission to attend the school of our choice. We were utterly stunned. The journalist had achieved more in those few days than we had in months.

The following day a letter arrived which confirmed that Christopher could begin school and that the issue of transport would be our responsibility. But we were absolutely delighted with the result and visited the press office to offer our sincere thanks for their support.

On March 15th 1993 Christopher became a pupil at Ebbw Vale and as agreed, Philip and I acted as escorts. However, within a few weeks more, the Education Department conceded that transport would be provided by the authority after all. The dilemma of locating a suitable school had finally been resolved.

CHAPTER THREE

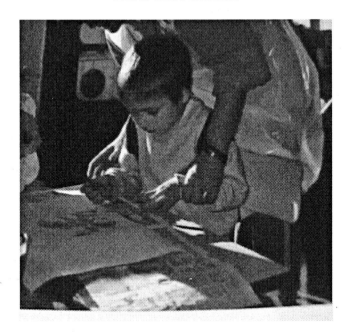

Christopher had been placed in a mixed ability class at school with children of similar age to his. He shared the class with approximately eight other pupils, which seems remarkably few, but this was typical of all of the special needs schools we had viewed. In addition to the smaller class size, the high staff ratio which consisted of a teacher and three classroom assistants meant that staff were able to give each pupil the maximum amount of attention and support they needed to reach their full potential.

Even so, it had taken many months for Christopher to adapt and settle to the new routine which school brought, as he had never been left with anyone until his recent placement at playgroup. He was very clingy and spent much of the first two terms pacing the classroom or pulling at the door, crying to return home and boarding the bus in the mornings had proven to be particularly traumatic for him.

It was also very stressful for us to visit the school for appointments because if he happened to notice that we were there he would scream and attack in an effort to come to us. Attempts to distract and comfort him were futile and the staff soon realised that it was necessary to maintain a safe distance between him and us at such times, to avoid the distress.

Improvements in the classroom were inevitably slow because of the extent of Christopher's learning delay and these entailed anything as basic as sitting for the duration of a short story to holding a loaded spoon at dinner time. Christopher was able to finger-feed with sandwiches, crisps etc; but he often chose to throw or crumble foods instead, as he enjoyed the texture of different foods against his skin. Nevertheless, any progress, no matter how small, was seen as an achievement and this in turn was exciting to learn of.

In addition to the regular timetable, pupils were taken on weekly outings and also enjoyed scheduled sessions of hydrotherapy, swimming and horse-riding. The latter was offered to different classes each term so that all of the children, who were able to support themselves on horse-back, eventually enjoyed this activity. Weekly outings ranged from visits to the local park in good weather, to trips to the shopping precinct which enhanced both social and life skills. Some of the more able pupils were able to purchase a favoured item for themselves, whilst other pupils could enjoy a similar treat which would be purchased by one of the classroom assistants from monies sent in from home.

Christopher's challenging behaviour was a source of concern from the very beginning and the school had concentrated all of their efforts into improving his communication ability. It was felt that Christopher's failure to make his needs and wishes understood was the primary cause of his frustration and resulting tantrums and it was hoped that by teaching him a way in which to communicate, he would not only be calmer, but also more accepting of learning.

A method of sign language called *Makaton* had already been adopted by the school and so this was slowly introduced. The staff noticed that although Christopher would wander around within minutes of the session beginning, he frequently glanced back and forth whilst the other children continued with the remainder of the session. He appeared to be interested by the use of hand gestures, but his understanding was hindered by his extensive disabilities.

In truth, Christopher's ability to play and amuse himself was also greatly impaired and he required high levels of interaction for much of the day. He would spend hours playing with sand and water and would push any object with wheels, but he completely ignored the numerous educational toys we had bought and they remained discarded in the toy box.

As much as 8 hours a day could be spent playing with preferred activities when he was in the mood, but as often as we felt that our presence alongside of him went unnoticed, if we happened to move and walk away, he would get to his feet and follow. Philip and I took it in turn to play and attempted to make interesting games out of the few toys which appealed to him. By elevating one end of the toy box lid a ramp could easily be created and when the gradient was varied, it demonstrated that the balls or cars would roll down at differing speeds. Using cars or balls in this way provided an ideal opportunity for the introduction of colours and numbers and games could be made out of asking what colour ball or car was rolling down the ramp and how fast it was going. This also gave Christopher the opportunity to hear a repetition of the various adjectives, nouns, verbs, etc. and made the games more fun.

It was whilst we were playing with a car one day that I noticed that Christopher would sometimes turn it around before pushing it back to me. At first I was just a little curious as to why he would do this, but as the game continued, I suddenly realised that the car was always returned to me in a forward-facing position. This immediately took my interest and so I decided to push the car to Christopher backward-facing, in a reverse-type position. He did not turn the car around on this occasion, but simply pushed it back to me. For the next few turns I pushed the car forward-facing and waited to see what would happen. Christopher turned the car every time before pushing it away.

I then decided to alternate the position of the car when I pushed it forwards and was stunned to observe Christopher turning it only when necessary, so that it was always returned forward-facing. He barely glanced at the car and to any casual observer, the rolling backwards and forth would have looked almost mechanical, but I suddenly realised with a smile that it was so much more.

Water held even more fascination for Christopher than any other toy or activity and he would happily spend upwards of an hour in the bath 2 – 3 times each day. He was still unable to climb into the bath himself and so one or both parents were needed to lift him in depending upon his mood. But as he played with so few toys, we were content to see the evident enjoyment on his face when the bath was filled and assumed that his sitting in the water would help prevent rashes from the pads he wore night and day.

Christopher showed no interest in playing with bath toys or water-wheels, but simply derived pleasure from splashing or trailing his hands through the warm, soapy suds. A plastic beaker was introduced so that water could be scooped up and poured back into the bath and we noticed that Christopher would hold his hand under the trickle of water when the beaker was tilted and emptied. He also loved the contents of the beaker to be poured over his shoulders and back as he sat quietly and the first time he took the beaker to copy this action, brought a smile to both our faces.

If Christopher loved to play with cars, then he enjoyed going out for drives just as much - as long as the car continued to move, that is. But it soon became apparent that he not only recognised red traffic lights, he also realised that whenever a light changed to red the car would cease moving. The result was always the same he would scream, bang on the window adjacent to him with his hands and bite the door directly below the window.

We learned that as traffic lights were situated on most roads, ignoring them was not an option and so we decided to make a game out of them instead. Christopher was asked, '*where's the green light?*' and when it finally showed we'd say, '*there it is; now we can go.*' This helped as a distraction, but did not completely alleviate the problem or the eventual protests if the wait was anything other than minimal.

Queues of traffic proved an even greater cause of distress as Christopher soon realised that when queues were ahead, the car would be prevented from moving. The tantrums would then be instantaneous and to avoid upsetting scenes, routes were eventually planned for drives in the country, where the car was rarely required to stop and he could relax and simply enjoy being out and about.

In addition to his dislike of slowing down or stopping in queues of traffic, Christopher also displayed distress whenever his buggy did the same. We began to realise that this was the probable cause of his tantrums whenever crowds of people were around him, as we would inevitably have to walk more slowly or even stop altogether. This realisation enabled us to make adjustments to our plans. We avoided shopping at busy times of the day and did not take him to environments which were typically crowded.

The summer holidays presented our family with more of a problem though as perspective destinations were inevitably going to be busier than usual. But, we decided that the solution to this dilemma was to arrive earlier than other visitors. We would plan an outing to the zoo, safari park or sea-side, ascertain the opening time, when relevant, and if Christopher awoke in a good mood we would then set off with the intention of arriving ahead of other people. By the time the crowds were about to descend upon us, he had generally become bored and was content to leave, but at least we managed day trips following this strategy.

Although we continued in our attempts to visit the family whenever behaviour permitted, it became a great strain and little enjoyment was ever derived out of what should have been a social time. Other homes were not safe environments for Christopher and we were constantly on our feet following him. Over time though, we realised that the type of mood he awoke in was typically a good indicator of the type of day we could expect from him. There were obviously some known trigger factors to behaviour deterioration which could alter the course of the day, but on the whole we discovered that it was a comparatively reliable way of determining a good day from a bad. This realisation enabled us to plan briefly ahead and to take advantage of calmer days. Visits and outings were scheduled for the occasions when Christopher was feeling more amiable and we found that he would often respond positively to such plans.

The months continued to pass by rapidly, but at home it was still impossible to leave him unsupervised in one room for chores to be completed in another, even for the briefest amount of time. Ordinary household objects which would not typically be considered to be dangerous suddenly became so with him chewing, pulling or touching them, but the stairs was undoubtedly our biggest concern.

The safety gate which had served its purpose well whilst he was a toddler was no match in strength for a larger-than-average five year old with severe behavioural problems and it had been ripped entirely off its hinges several months earlier. Fortunately, Christopher showed only a mild interest in the stairs, but we were always on our guard and aware that his love of water might eventually lead him to venture up to the bathroom.

The kitchen was also another area of concern as the door could no longer be left open whilst food was being prepared, as Christopher had grown too tall for protection guards to serve any purpose. He could easily reach saucepans, kettles and throw objects which were placed on the back of work-surfaces and so he was not allowed in the room. However, if one parent was alone whilst cooking then the door could not be closed against him either, as he needed to be watched closely. This resulted in our decision to build and install a stable-type door to replace the original. This prevented Christopher from accessing the kitchen, but enabled us to see what he was doing and also allowed him to watch us from the safety of the hallway so that he didn't feel completely excluded.

Since the deterioration of his sleeping pattern at 18 months, we had been unable to re-establish a night time routine and Christopher typically ran around the lounge until exhaustion finally got the better of him, which was usually between the hours of 3.00am – 5.00am. We would wait until he was sleeping heavily before carrying him upstairs and if this was timed just right, he would remain asleep when he was placed in bed. However, if we misjudged how heavily he was sleeping, our lifting would wake him, and as exhausted as he was, he would struggle to free himself and continue to run around for a few hours more.

However, despite his obvious exhaustion and the minimal amount of time which he spent sleeping, he still continued to wake up at frequent intervals and attempts to settle him back to sleep were impossible. Occasionally he spent the entire night running around or pacing the floor, fighting off sleep altogether.

In an attempt to allow one parent to get some sleep we decided that it would be beneficial for us to take it in turns at the *night-shift*, but this proved to be impractical from the start. It was not easy to fall asleep whilst Christopher spent hours screaming and banging the wooden banister and it was even harder to remain asleep if we actually managed to drop off in the first place. The noise was deafening in our own home and we were very aware that our neighbours must have been subjected to as many disturbed nights as we were. We frequently apologised for the disturbance and although they were very sympathetic, our concerns for their welfare added to the stress that we were already under.

If the nights were exhausting then there was no improvement to be found in the days, with Christopher continually pacing the floor or running around. He had always on occasions bitten the back of his wrist and any sleeves which covered it could be destroyed within minutes, when he was in that type of mood. But, he had recently begun to lift the waist-bands of clothing into his mouth to chew and on particularly bad days, he would destroy as many as 3 tee-shirts or jumpers. Ironically, although he still crawled and led down to play, it was only necessary to replace trousers when they no longer fitted, but the same could not be said for the furniture.

Sofas and chairs were frequently replaced with family cast-offs or second-hand substitutes, as Christopher would either bite the material off the arms to expose the foam beneath, or break the springs and wooden frame by running and dropping down heavily onto them. Bedding was also mouthed and chewed and crockery was thrown at mealtimes and since Christopher had been able to lift and throw the television from the cabinet, both had been replaced. A new cabinet with doors on the front was purchased, which protected the new television and we were relieved to discover that it worked as a deterrent.

…But as desperate as our financial concerns could be, the first time Christopher passed his beaker to request a drink, we were completely elated. It was a basic gesture, but it was one that had been instigated by Christopher himself and the request was easily understood. Soon he also realised that by passing a plastic plate, we would understand this to mean a request for food and so, communication using basic objects of reference, had began. We were optimistic that the range of objects being used could be improved upon as Christopher grew older and readily accepted the offer of the involvement of a psychologist, hoping that any advice given, might also involve strategies on how to manage problem behaviours.

In November 1993 our son Craig was involved in a road accident and sadly died. Christopher's behaviour altered in the months that followed and he wandered around the house as if searching for his brother. Staff noticed a difference in him at school and it became apparent that he realised something had happened, although how much of what he understood, could only be guessed at.

But whatever the level of his understanding, it was clear that he felt anxious when anyone left the room and we soon became accustomed to seeing Christopher tailing each of us around in turn until he was satisfied that we were where we should be.

For Michael, it was a traumatic and confusing time and although he had the ability to communicate his feelings, he refused to do so. Philip and I also had great difficulty in our grief, afraid of upsetting everyone else and hoping that by not talking about the accident, it made it less real. It was stupid, but the most unexpected and devastating event had happened to our family and none of us knew how to accept it and finally, how to come to terms with it

. . . .

CHAPTER FOUR

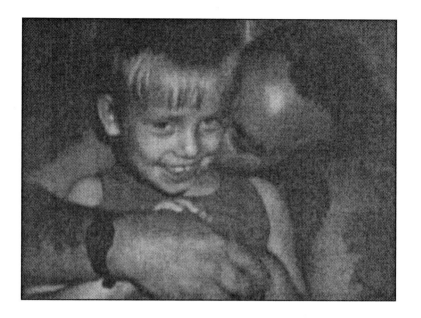

Philip with Christopher aged 7 years

Christopher continued to make slow but steady progress with communicating his needs and in addition to being able to request drinks or food, he had now also learnt to associate a bunch of keys with being taken out in the car. He had evidently noticed his father carrying the keys whenever we went out for a drive and realised that they were in someway connected with our using the car.

The first time that he took the keys off the hook near the front door and presented them to his father, we were a little confused as to what he actually wanted, but then something suddenly *clicked* into place and we understood. Philip accepted the offered keys, placed the harness on Christopher and we went out for the drive which he had requested.

He began to make other connections with our going out for a drive. He was much more adept visually and noticed that before we went outside, the television and fire were turned off and shoes were placed on his feet. He soon learned to touch the television or fire-guard and even collected and presented us with shoes to request a drive. The shoes were not always his, but the item was still meant to convey his desire to go out and we understood it to mean as much.

Alternatively, if he wished to go outside in the garden to play, he would go to the back door and either touch it, or pull the handle in an attempt to open it. Philip or I would then unlock the door and ensure that he reached the bottom tier of the garden in safety. He loved to be outside in the fresh air and the garden was the only place out of doors where he did not have to be restrained in his buggy. It was lovely to watch him walking or running freely, it was just sad that the garden was such a small one and did not provide the space that he evidently needed.

Nevertheless, as he loved to be out in the open air we had done our best over the years to provide garden toys and equipment which would keep him both stimulated and interested, whilst at the same time being fun for his brothers. A large sand-pit had proven to be one of the best purchases as he would spend hours trailing his fingers through the grains or flicking handfuls up into the air and watching it fall. In warmer weather his paddling pool was inflated and filled with water and he either sat in it, or against it, splashing wildly. We often ended up as drenched as he did but he loved the sensation of the water cascading over his arms, legs and face.

Lastly, we bought the children a swing set, but soon discovered that although Christopher would sit on the junior swing quite happily, he would not hold on to the chains to prevent himself from falling off the seat. We placed his hands on the chains and covered them with ours to demonstrate what he needed to do, but irrespective of how often this action was repeated, he would drop his own hands down to his sides once ours was removed. It was difficult to know if Christopher did not *want* to hold the chains or did not understand that he *needed* to, but whatever the reason, the result would be the same so he was taken off the swing and placed on the carriage-type one instead.

The design of the carriage swing made it far safer for him to use as he did not have to hold on if he preferred not to. Two enclosed seats with raised backs and sides faced each other, whilst a platform was attached some short distance beneath the bottom of the seats. Christopher loved this new toy and on fine days he would spend hours smiling whilst Philip and I took it in turns to push him back and forth.

It was whilst he was walking in the garden one day that I noticed a small group of children congregating around the fence, but it wasn't until I drew nearer that I realised that they were teasing him.

The fence was over 6 feet in height but it was the design of it which was proving to be the problem. Vertical slats were attached to a large rectangular frame and it was between the slats, in the spaces the design provided, that the children had slid a stick through with the intention of hurting him.

Christopher was giggling and completely unaware of the negative attention which he was receiving but I was upset and I pondered over how we could prevent similar incidents from recurring. I decided that as the gaps in the fence were providing an opportunity for children to touch or hurt him, then the solution was to block up the spaces with wooden panels. If the panels were then stained with the same colour fence-life as the existing fence, it would blend in and not look out of place.

As we needed 4 panels and required them to be 4 feet in height by 8 feet in length we decided to purchase them from the local salvage merchant to cut down on the cost. They were stained on one side and later screwed onto the existing fence with the stain facing outwards. I had originally intended to repeat the same process on the insides of the panels too, but when I looked at the large boards facing into the garden I suddenly had the idea to paint them. I had always loved drawing and painting and knowing that Christopher loved to watch Disney cartoons and was particularly fond of The Jungle Book, I decided to paint a different scene from the film on each of the four panels and whilst the rain replaced the warmth of the sunshine, I carried my paints and brushes underneath the tarpaulin that now protected the fence and set to work.

I used chalk to draw the pictures and filled in the details with gloss paint so that it would be protected against the weather and just two days later, the paintings were complete. We stood back from the panels to study each one in turn and were absolutely delighted with the result. Not only did the bottom tier of the garden now protect Christopher from unwanted attention, but it also resembled a nursery play area.

The psychologist had made several visits by this time and had advised us to use single words or stinted sentences whenever we spoke to Christopher as it was apparent that he still did not understand speech. This particular piece of advice had proved invaluable and with months of daily repetition it had enabled him to recognise the words drink, food and car. It hadn't been too difficult for Christopher to make a connection between *eating* and the word *food* as he had always enjoyed his meals. But the appetite, which had been consistent since he was a baby, slowly began to alter and over time he rarely ate a typical quantity of food, but went from one extreme to another.

There were occasions when his appetite grew so large that he devoured astonishing amounts of food, often resulting in him eating so much that he would vomit. As this phase could last for days, weeks or even months at a time, it became necessary to limit his food intake and to substitute typical foods with lower-fat alternatives to prevent health problems. Even so, it was difficult to keep his weight within a normal range during this eating phase or to offer distractions, as his only interest at such times would be in determining what the next meal would consist of.

However, there were also occasions when he would stop requesting meals altogether and did not appear to notice that he was hungry, despite having eaten only tiny amounts of food all day. We prepared favourite foods in the hope of tempting him and when one snack or meal was refused, another took its place, but Christopher was stubborn and continued to ignore our efforts.

Again, the phase of refusing to eat could last for days, weeks or even months at a time and it was distressing to see the alarming weight loss it resulted in, as the slim child was slowly replaced by an even skinnier substitute. Christopher's tee-shirts and jumpers began to hang on him and the elasticised trousers which he always wore for comfort would fall down over the bulk of his incontinence pad. The tops looked strange and outsized but they did not need replacing if they had not been bitten. However, the trousers became so noticeably large that new ones had become a necessity.

The doctor was consulted about the problem and a prescription for drink supplements was issued. The drinks contained a variety of vitamins and calories which prevented Christopher from becoming dangerously underweight and it was hoped that the added vitamins would encourage normal eating to resume. As he was very fussy with the types and varieties of food and drink which he would try, we were relieved to notice that they were accepted because the fruit flavours were fortunately very similar to his standard drink.

The different eating phases came and went at regular intervals but during the non-eating stage, it was incredibly upsetting to sit eating a meal in front of Christopher, whilst he refused all offers of foods and snacks. Inevitably we felt very guilty to be eating our own meals, although it had to be admitted that the lack of food did not appear to have any noticeable effect on him. He slept as badly as ever and his energy levels were equally as high as they had always been.

It was whilst Christopher was running around at school in the clumsy way we now associated with him, that he stumbled and fell, hitting his mouth in the process. It wasn't a particularly nasty fall, but when the dentist visited the school some months later he noticed that an abscess had formed above the two front teeth which had been knocked.

The dentist then made a home visit where we were advised that a referral had been made for the teeth to be extracted. Furthermore, our concerns about how Christopher would cope were intensified when we realised that the procedure was going to be completed in hospital, under general anaesthetic and not at a surgery. A few days later the senior consultant also made a home visit so that he could assess Christopher and although he was in a good mood we were advised that it would be necessary to sedate him before he arrived at the hospital. I stressed that a previous attempt at sedation had not worked for an in-depth hearing test when he had been a toddler, but the consultant assured me that it would be successful.

The medication was to be given in 2 oral syringes 1 hour before we left for the hospital on the day of surgery. We were advised that it would initially make Christopher very drowsy and by the time we were ready to leave the house to keep our appointment, he would be sleeping soundly and would need to be carried out to the car.

The day of the appointment arrived and whilst Michael and Philip restrained him as best they could, I placed the syringe into his open mouth and administered the first dose. Legs and arms flayed wildly as he attempted to free himself, but we persevered and managed to repeat the process once again before allowing him to run from us and calm down.

As the time of our departure drew near, we watched for signs that the medication was beginning to work, but Christopher was as hyperactive as ever and did not become even mildly drowsy. We collected his bag which contained enough pads, drinks, toys, etc; for the hours we were expecting to be at the hospital and taking his hands we walked out to the car.

He giggled during the twenty minute journey and we were thankful that he had awoken in a good mood. There was no doubt in our minds that his behaviour would deteriorate over the course of the day, but at least for the moment he was relaxed and fairly amiable.

Inside the hospital three nurses were awaiting our arrival and whilst one of them asked me questions about Christopher's general health, the other two attempted to carry out the pre-operative examinations. This task became increasingly difficult to complete as Christopher had began to grab everything within arms reach. Philip and Michael did their best to prevent him from doing so but with desks, shelves and cupboards covered by equipment or papers, they fought a losing battle.

As he became more vocal in his protests, arrangements were made for him to be placed in a separate room and Philip and Michael were directed to one which was situated away from the main ward, whilst I remained with the nurse to answer the remaining questions without further disruption.

When I joined them a short time later I discovered that the anaesthetist was already present and insisting that additional sedation be given. Christopher had been scheduled for the first appointment of the day but the procedure could not be completed until he had succumbed to the medication and at that time he was very obviously wide awake, distressed and aggressive. A nurse entered the room carrying an oral syringe and we were asked to take Christopher out of his buggy so that he could be restrained on the bed and whilst four pairs of hands attempted to hold him he fought ferociously, resulting in the nurse being kicked.

Finally, we were left alone for the sedation to take effect, but Christopher showed little signs of any weariness as he continued to run around the room, pulling at the taps in the sink and attempting to dismantle the medical equipment which was housed there. As more time elapsed he became increasingly distressed and nurses took to peering through the pane of glass which was situated in the door, in preference to opening it and actually entering the room.

An hour later it was obvious that the additional sedative had not had any effect and so the nurses decided to administer a further dose. He was restrained and fought again as attempts to place the syringe in his mouth were made and we were further distressed to notice that he had blood around his lips and tongue. He was again held so that the source of the bleeding could be located and with relief we were advised that the syringe must have scraped against his gum and grazed it. Still, Christopher had always looked to us to comfort and support him and our part in his distress made us feel like traitors.

The procedure of restraining him to administer yet more doses of sedation was continued on 3 more occasions without any noticeable effect and when the anaesthetist made another visit to the room to request that he be subjected to further doses, Philip finally refused and we were left alone.

A few more hours passed by and we were relieved to discover that he was eventually becoming weary. He climbed onto the bed and I lay alongside of him, cuddling him in the nook of my arm for what seemed an age. Finally, the door was pushed open but when I attempted to climb off the bed, I was asked to remain with him whilst he was wheeled to the theatre. As we approached our destination I began to lower my legs to the floor when he suddenly leapt off the bed and attempted to abscond. The theatre staff was quick to react and restrained him for the final time and as the gas mask was placed over his face, it was with relief I noticed that the effect was immediate. The extractions were completed some 4 hours later than first scheduled but at least it was over and done with.

However, following Christopher's experience at hospital, his behaviour deteriorated to an alarming extent and our general practitioner made a referral to the paediatrician. The severity of the behaviours we described and duration of attacks led to a further referral for Christopher to be seen by a psychiatrist and he was finally prescribed anti-psychotic medication.

We had always been completely against such medicines as we felt that they were the easy way out, but we were exhausted and terrified of losing our son to residential care as we were not able to cope with the severity of the attacks. Christopher had always presented us with challenging behaviour but these outbursts were unlike anything we had ever witnessed before. The look of hatred in his eyes altered his facial expression beyond all recognition and at times I saw no part of Christopher in the child that looked back at me at all.

That period of time saw Philip and I reach an all time low as we realised the full implications of Christopher's behaviour and of what the future would hold. Attacks were sudden, occurred without provocation and once started, continued for 8 – 12 hours. But for all of the difficulties, he was our son and we loved him.

....

CHAPTER FIVE

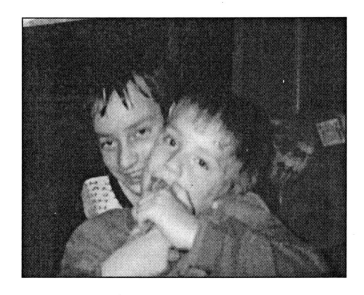

Michael with Christopher aged 9 years

It had been over a year since Christopher had visited the hospital for his teeth extractions and his behaviour had at last began to settle and things had returned to a different kind of normal. However, his moods were less predictable than they had previously been and calm behaviours in the morning were no longer a reliable indication of the type of day we could expect from him, with *or* without triggers.

The ferocious outbursts of aggression had once again subsided but the psychologist continued to have input and it was during one of our discussions that I realised her understanding of his behavioural patterns was somewhat misunderstood, despite our best efforts to detail them.

I realised that the behaviours were inconsistent and whilst on one occasion a distraction or removal from a situation *might* be possible, during times of *higher* levels of aggression, the same approach would be rendered useless. Yet to admit that the approach might work at one time, and not on another, sounded contradictory and needed further explanation.

I decided to detail the different types of behaviour which Christopher presented with and place them into *stages*, or *levels* of aggression. Level 1 described the calmest Christopher could be and explained that at this level he would be amiable, pleasant and easily distractible. His concentration was at its best and he would often be very loving, climbing onto our laps to offer kisses and cuddles.

If he awoke in this type of mood it would continue all day and probably even for several days or weeks at a time. We would not expect to experience any challenging behaviour, but he might throw or grab in fun, which would often be accompanied by mischievous giggling.

At level 2 he often displayed much of the previous behaviours *but* the probability of him attacking without provocation would be present. At this type of level, outbursts could leave mild bruising and cuts, but they were manageable by those who knew him. Types of behaviours which could be anticipated were biting, nail-gouging, hair pulling, slapping, punching and throwing, but Christopher could still be distracted and outbursts were not prolonged.

He would also present with self-injurious behaviours, specifically biting the back of his wrist, but we typically wound bandage around this area until it was of sufficient thickness to offer protection. Failing to do so would result in infections and areas of missing skin and, as with the previous level, if Christopher awoke in this type of mood, it would typically last for days or even weeks at a time.

Level 3 described the behaviours which we experienced following the hospital appointment and detailed serious prolonged attacks which lasted for 8 - 12 hours in duration. At this level his strength was phenomenal; outbursts were explosive and people-orientated. He would throw and self-injure, but only as a second resort. His main intention in this type of level was to injure others.

Bites would result in infections and mass bruising and clothing would be literally ripped away as Christopher used the material to pull others towards his mouth. Hair would be pulled out from scalps and skin would be left scarred where his nails had torn into it. There was no distraction from attacks and Christopher paused only long enough to regulate his breathing. He would sweat profusely, and often be very vocal during outbursts, screaming or grunting as he ran forward. There was never any warning of stage 3 attacks. He could be offering cuddles and kisses on the numerous occasions he awoke during the night, only to finally awake in this type of mood. But this highest level of aggression was only displayed occasionally and following sleep – behaviour *never* deteriorated to this level from level 2.

I recalled the previous year and how the different levels of aggression had manifested themselves on a daily basis. Christopher had been calm and loving one moment only to lunge in frenzied attacks the next and we had constantly needed to be on our guard to avoid serious injuries. It was true that his behaviour could deteriorate with triggers, but *never* to this extent and *never* before had level 3 type behaviours mixed with the other levels in the same day.

I scrolled down the screen, reading the behavioural descriptors and was satisfied that they provided a clearer understanding of the different levels of aggression which Christopher presented. I hoped that the psychologist would now understand why, on certain occasions, the same approach would simply prove to be ineffective and on offering a copy to place in his file, I was pleased to note that it did.

It was during this particular visit that the psychologist stated that Christopher suffered from intermittent noise and visual intolerance. She explained that having studied him in school and home environments it had become apparent that he experienced this type of sensory overload, which was a common difficulty in people with autism.

This information intrigued me as I had never before heard of *sensory overload*, but as far as the issue of noise intolerance was concerned it explained why he would sometimes place the palms of his hands over his ears and scream. Noises did not have to be loud for him to do this, but apparently any sounds would be amplified during affected days, much like sitting next to a speaker on full volume. This also explained why the same volume of sounds on one day could excite or be ignored by him, only to cause him great distress on another day.

We immediately agreed with the psychologist's diagnosis of noise intolerance as it made sense of his behaviour, but we were not so sure about the issue of him being affected visually and asked for the reasons behind this assumption. The psychologist stated that she had seen Christopher covering his eyes in much the same way as he covered his ears and explained that he had also used blankets and other items in school to do this.

We suddenly realised that he also did this at home, but as he displayed many strange mannerisms, which were again characteristic of autism, we had assumed that face and head covering were simply more of the same. We were fascinated and wanted to know more. The psychologist asked if we had ever seen television footage of a crowded shopping precinct speeded up and explained that on affected days it was likely that Christopher processed visual data in much the same way. Either types of intolerance would understandably increase the risk of distress and aggression, so we were advised that strategies needed to be in place for the times when he was affected.

Ear-plugs could be purchased from a sports shop to be used during noise intolerant days and she advised that we continue to keep him away from noisy and crowded places. Minimising noises around the home as best we could was also necessary by having the volume of the television, radio, etc, on low and removing toys with *light* and *sound* functions during these phases.

With no room to retreat to downstairs, we were advised to leave a blanket or towel around to enable Christopher to cover his head during days when he suffered from visual intolerance. He needed to feel calm and relaxed and the material would help to block out what the psychologist referred to as *visual noise*. The strategies were not ideal but at least they would help ease the situation a little and we were grateful to have input from such a knowledgeable source.

At school, staff had also endured a difficult year as concerns about his aggression had increased along with his size and during the annual review the Special Educational Needs officer requested that we visit 2 schools which specialised in autism. We were also asked if we would consider sending Christopher to residential school in Birmingham or Somerset, but although we agreed to visit the other schools we immediately refused the suggestion of residential schooling.

Following the review, arrangements were first made for Philip and me to visit the school in Cardiff which was situated some 30 miles away. The school itself was lovely and the classes were made up of a small number of children with varying degrees of autism. Some of the pupils also presented with challenging behaviour although none of them to the same extent as Christopher.

The rooms were designed with considerable detail and in addition to the existing tables, further ones ran along the walls, which were partitioned off in cubicle-fashion. The partitions enabled students to concentrate on individual tasks with the teacher or classroom assistant, without any visual distractions from anywhere else in the room.

We were intrigued to learn that some of the children without speech, or poor speech had been using a method of communication called PECS. This we learned stood for Picture, Exchange, Communication, System. It was an ingenious idea whereby children selected appropriate pictures on cards to communicate their wishes or needs. The card could be made specifically to tailor individual requirements, such as a like of ballet, bowling, visits to cinema, etc, but pictures could also eventually be used to visually detail a timetable for children.

On the most basic level the pupils were taught how to offer a card in exchange for a favourite snack, activity, etc. For instance, if the favoured item was a packet of crisps, then the child would sit at the opposite end of the table to a teacher and a PEC card would be placed in front of the child. The teacher would take a crisp between a finger and thumb and hold it at shoulder level, whilst at the same time holding their free hand outwards.

Initially, an assistant would help the child to pick up the PEC card off the table and to place it in the open hand of the teacher, much like a ticket. Once the card was handed over, the teacher would pass a single crisp to the child before placing the card back onto the table for the procedure to be repeated. Once the packet of crisps had been eaten the session would end, but 20-plus exchanges could be made per session and if a further 4 sessions were scheduled each day, the repetition would aid quicker learning of the system.

When this first stage was mastered and the child could place the card into the teacher's hand without prompting or assistance, they were taught how to learn to differentiate between the pictures on the cards. This opened up a whole new way of communicating without the use of speech or the written word. After all, if anyone handed over a card containing a picture of a burger and chips in any café or shop, the request would be obvious.

We were very impressed with both the school and the system and were equally as impressed to discover that the same method of communication was being used at the second autism school which we visited in Bridgend, some 45 miles away from home.

This school was set out differently to the first in that the children were divided into rooms on the ground and first floor, depending upon their ages. The ground floor rooms were beautifully decorated and visually stimulating, reminding me of nursery and infant days. There were a wide range of toys and activities to cater for the varying abilities of the children and an impressive music room housed some equally impressive instruments and equipment, but the part of the school which stole my heart was the outside play area. This was a superb mixture of safety rubber-flooring and space, which the younger children appeared to love and we were fortunate enough to be granted a few moments to watch before we were shown to the first floor.

The rooms upstairs were situated on either side of a wide corridor and as we made our way along we noticed that the door in which we had just entered was being locked behind us. This was to prevent any of the pupils from absconding and endangering themselves. We were immediately struck by the lack of colour on the upper floor in contrast to the ground floor. An occasional poster adorned the walls but for the most part it was white and sterile looking, although not in an unpleasant way.

Inside the school, we noticed that there were hook-and-eye type fasteners on the tops of all of the doors and these were secured whenever we exited through them. We also noted that the cupboards and other large furnishings were bolted to the walls in various rooms to prevent them from being upturned or thrown.

As we walked around the school we realised that we hadn't seen any evidence of a lift to take pupils from the ground to the first floor. We had used the large stairway which was situated near the reception area to reach the upper level and could only assume that the pupils at the school had the ability to use the stairs in safety.

As lovely as both schools were the reason for our visits had resulted from the severity of aggression which Christopher could present with. …And even though both schools had pupils with similar diagnosis to his, neither had experience of similar behaviours and in most instances, outbursts typically lasted no more than ten minutes and was *significantly* milder. This being the case, there was no more reason to suspect that the staff here would be any more able to cope with severe outbursts than staff at the present school.

More worrying still was the distance both schools were from home and the amount of traffic and queues which Christopher would be waiting in on a daily basis. Waiting in queues of traffic each day would result in behavioural deterioration whatever the original mood type he awoke in, so having weighed up the pros and cons of changing schools, we decided not to proceed any further.

Following the visits we advised the head teacher that we wished for Christopher to remain at the school, but we also mentioned the exciting new communication system we had seen and asked if selected members of staff could visit the schools to learn how it was taught. It would be a fantastic opportunity, not only for pupils with a diagnosis of autism, but for any pupil experiencing difficulties with communication.

After all, Christopher had made no progress with using sign language as it was too complex for him to relate to and we were positive that some of the less able pupils must also be experiencing similar difficulties. Our suggestion was greeted with some mild interest but we were disappointed to learn that PECS was not introduced to the pupils.

Although the situation at school was undoubtedly a worry we were soon to be distracted by concerns nearer to home. Philip had fallen in the car park during the recent snow fall and sustained a spiral break to his ankle and lower leg. The break had required surgery and he had remained in hospital to have pins inserted to support the fractures. As I was unable to lift and carry Christopher upstairs on my own I was left with little option than to bring blankets down and make beds up on the sofa.

Philip was discharged from hospital a week later, but he remained in plaster for the following six weeks and was unable to assist in carrying him upstairs during this time. He was also unable to manage the stairs himself and so each night I hauled the double mattress down into the lounge, with enough blankets to make up beds for the three of us.

Christopher had always resisted being taken to bed and having slept in the lounge for almost two months, we were unable to re-establish the previous routine which had, at best, always been unstable to begin with. So, with reluctance we continued with the new sleeping arrangements. But although the situation was far from ideal, we were exhausted by our years of struggling upstairs with him each night and afraid of the injuries our dropping him would result in.

. . . .

CHAPTER SIX

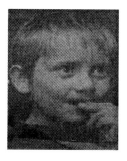

Christopher aged 10 years

As Christopher became larger and his ability to manage steps did not improve, stumbles on the stairs were an everyday occurrence. Mostly they had resulted in nothing more than mild scrapes and bruising, but lately we had been concerned by the potential of more serious injuries.

On one occasion he had been holding my hand as we walked from the bathroom having enjoyed one of his usual water-play sessions. He was in a pleasant enough mood and was walking nicely beside me until we reached the top of the stairs. Michael had just returned home and was in the process of running up the stairs when Christopher suddenly became very excited and jumped off the top step towards him.

I recall how I watched in horror as his hand slipped from mine and Michael fought to prevent them both from tumbling down the stairs, by gripping the banister as they fell against it. As I ran towards them I grabbed Michael's free arm and helped him to his feet and although Christopher had found the whole episode amusing, I shook as I realised just how lucky they had both been.

On another occasion I had been leading Christopher down stairs when he suddenly lunged forward to attack me. We had probably reached about halfway when this happened and although I was holding the banister with my free hand, which slowed down our fall, my left foot remained on the step and took the weight of our bodies as we fell forward onto the hard floor of the hall. A serious sprain and suspected tendon damage left me out of action for weeks but I was relieved that it hadn't been more serious as it could easily have resulted in broken limbs or worse.

In some respects his increase in size meant that he was more prone to falling as his feet were the same length as each step and always hung over the edges. But although stumbles and falls were a regular occurrence, he was not in any way afraid of using the stairs and in his naivety had recently begun to take more of an interest in them.

Christopher's tendency to drop to the ground and refusal to walk had also worsened over the years and he would attack those attempting to help him to his feet if he wished to remain where he was sitting or lying. He looked exactly like an out-sized toddler having a tantrum and, this, in effect, is precisely what he was.

If he was walking with others he would also attack in an effort to break free and with no awareness of danger, roads remained a constant concern. His strength was unsurpassed when he was pulling to free himself and staff at school had now automatically begun to use a wheelchair to take him to and from the bus, as this was the safest and quickest method. An assessment had also provided him with his own wheelchair for use at home and although this meant that we could travel around in safety, it did not solve the difficulties we encountered when taking him to and from the car-park.

The house which we had moved into when Christopher was just 2 months old had been built on a slope and there were several concrete steps which we had to negotiate leading down to and up from the property. The concrete slabs which overhang each step may not have posed too much of a problem whilst he was a toddler in a buggy, but he was now several stones in weight and could no longer be lifted safely.

It was possible to ascend the steps in relative safety *if* Christopher was not aggressive and *if* he was prepared to walk, but descending steps with him pulling forward or attacking, was simply horrendous and had resulted in numerous injuries and hospital treatment to family members. During the occasions when he would not co-operate it had therefore become necessary to carry him between 2 people – one parent taking the weight of his upper body and the other taking the weight of his legs.

It had become a common sight for neighbours to see him being carried in this way whilst screaming and kicking to free himself, oblivious to the dangers his succeeding would result in. But although this strategy was far from ideal, it was the safest method we had devised at that time and at least it enabled us to reach the car.

We were experiencing enormous mobility and safety difficulties, in and around the home but although these difficulties were apparent to neighbours and friends, it had taken many years to establish this fact with the Housing Department. Furthermore, despite our request for an assessment to determine if Christopher would be eligible for a bungalow, we had originally been placed on a list to move house.

It was true that a house move would have solved the problems we experienced when using the steps which led to the car-park, but any house we moved into would still have stairs inside and it had been a long struggle for us to find a way of making our dilemma better understood. All of the professionals who had become involved with Christopher had written to the Director of Housing over the years. Each had stressed the safety and mobility issues we experienced, as a direct result of the severity of his learning delay coupled with his behavioural difficulties. But it wasn't until we were offered, and refused another 3-bedroom house, that our difficulties were taken seriously.

I wrote to the Director to explain our reasons for the refusal and also provided details of the accidents and injuries we had all sustained when attempting to use stairs with Christopher. I explained that there were many occasions during the day when we resorted to carrying him – often with him struggling to free himself – and that when we actually managed to get him where we needed him, as he was mobile, there was no guarantee that he would stay.

The situation was difficult enough at present but neither Philip nor I could envisage carrying him around when he was a teenager, in just a few years time, or warding off attacks in such a dangerous environment. I ended my letter by enquiring who was to be held accountable if one of us was seriously injured as a direct result of the Council's failure to provide the assessment we had requested. I posted the letter but admittedly held out little hope of our request being taken seriously. But, a few days later we were thrilled to receive a response advising that the Occupational Therapist would be assessing Christopher to evaluate his needs.

The assessment itself was straight forward and we were relieved to learn that he did in fact meet the necessary criteria for bungalow eligibility. However, instead of placing us on a waiting list for a bungalow as anticipated, the Director planned to have an extension built in the back garden, which would contain a bedroom and bathroom for Christopher's use. We were utterly dismayed and again stressed that we were encountering as many difficulties in negotiating the concrete steps *outside* of the house as we did coping with the stairs *inside*. But our concerns were completely ignored and arrangements were made for a surveyor to view the property.

As the weeks passed by we realised the implications of any extension being built. There would be workmen traipsing through the house with no understanding of Christopher's problems – leaving doors open, tools and other equipment scattered around, etc, not to mention the inevitable noise.

There was no front garden, the door opened straight onto a pathway and so the extension was planned for the back garden. This meant that the lounge, which currently overlooked the back garden, would be thrown into almost total darkness when the large window was removed and blocked up with bricks, so that it could become the new bedroom wall. There were plans for a small window to be fitted at the side of the house, but three quarters of the room would receive no natural daylight whatsoever as the lounge would then be situated between the kitchen and the extension.

As the extension would take up most of the garden, the Director planned to move the fence so that the end of the garden was extended onto the pathway. This would provide Christopher with roughly the same amount of outside space that he currently had. But with the removal of the pathway, our neighbours would have to wheel their refuse bins down concrete steps, onto the main road below the houses, up a steep hill and back into the car-park for emptying each week.

The route would be impractical, if not impossible with full bins. …And we hadn't even begun to consider how our own bin would reach the car-park for emptying, but the final plan was to brick up the bottom of the stairs and fit a door which would prevent Christopher from gaining access to them. *If* the property had been built on a flat surface then we would have been overjoyed at the prospect of an extension, but there were no plans for the steps outside and any perspective work would have horrendous consequences for Christopher.

Eventually the surveyor came to the house to complete his assessment. We were distressed by the continuous delays but could not help feel relief when the subsequent report stated that as the garden would require huge amounts of concrete to level off the extensive gradient, an extension would not be feasible. This meant that with no other option available Christopher was finally placed on the waiting list for a bungalow and because of the known risks he was also given priority status.

With the housing issue looking more promising than ever before, family life was still difficult, but at least we now saw light at the end of the tunnel. We were also as delighted when Social Services managed to arrange 2-hours of weekly respite which was to be supplied by 2 support workers. There were conditions attached to us receiving this service, being that if Christopher was displaying any signs of aggression we were to contact the social worker and cancel the session, but having waited several years without success to receive family-based respite, we were simply happy to be offered any practical help at all.

The support workers were lovely but deciding where to take a child who did not cope around people was proving to be extremely difficult. During the warmer weather he could be taken for rides in his wheelchair, as long as the areas being visited were not overly noisy and people could not pass too near him.

But, any loud noises could aggravate his intolerance and trigger problem behaviours and if people passed within reach of the wheelchair, it was more than probable that he would pull them over. Smaller children would be particularly vulnerable given his increased size and strength. In any event, he did not always cope around adults, but he had never been particularly fond of other children, whom he tended to knock down or attack.

This had always created major problems during visits from the extended family and although we had long reached the stage where we could go into other people's homes, visits from others had diminished, with only my sisters now making any effort to keep in contact. Even so, with only a lounge, kitchen and toilet downstairs, it was sometimes necessary to turn visitors away if Christopher was particularly aggressive, as although the kitchen was typically used because of the safety of the stable-door, visitors still had to walk through the small hallway first and this in itself, caused us difficulties.

It was necessary to restrain Christopher when anyone entered the house, this was partly to prevent him from pushing past visitors to abscond and also because he could attack. But this meant that it was almost always necessary to have two parents present for visitors – one to restrain and one to open the door and usher people inside. Christopher could then wander around the lounge, but if anyone wanted to use the lavatory, the whole process of restraining needed to be completed again and also, when visitors left.

During calmer days, visits from my sisters did not create a significant problem as they knew him and could see themselves into the kitchen. And of course, if he was particularly good, there were still occasions when we could still sit in the lounge. But, if I was alone, or if he was very aggressive, there were times when I simply called through the letter-box to tell them of the situation and they left.

Over time Christopher became more relaxed with the support workers and even began to look forward to his outings. He knew that if his bag was being prepared that he would be going out and he often smiled and giggled in anticipation of the doorbell ringing. It was lovely to see that he was coping so well with this change in his routine and we hoped that things would continue to improve.

There were occasions when we had to cancel sessions and also occasions when he was returned home early without warning, but we hoped that as time went on and the workers became more confident with their management of him these times would lessen and respite would be more stable.

....

CHAPTER SEVEN

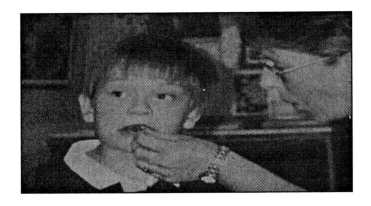

In November 1999 I suddenly found myself awoken in the early hours of the morning to find Christopher sitting bolt upright on the mattress, staring ahead. He was trembling slightly and looked frightened, as if he had been having some kind of nightmare. I wasn't sure what he could have dreamt about that had scared him so much, because I was unaware of anything that he was bothered by during the day, but he had evidently been frightened by something.

I quickly sat up, draped an arm around his shoulder and spoke in what I hoped was a reassuring manner. The episode only lasted for a minute at most before he sighed and leaned back against his pillow, instantly falling asleep. I watched as his breathing became more regular and assured that everything was now fine, I also leaned back down and fell asleep.

Philip and I discussed the incident the following morning and when no similar episodes recurred the following nights, we decided that he must have had a nightmare and thought no more about it. However, in the week leading up to Christmas Christopher experienced three more of these *episodes* and so we decided to mention them to the paediatrician during our next visit. After I had described the incidents in detail the paediatrician diagnosed *night terrors* and advised that he would eventually grow out of having them. She assured us that they were not dangerous in any way and were quite common in young children.

Neither Philip nor I had ever heard of *night terrors* before, but when we later discussed the diagnosis with members of the family, we discovered that one of my nephews also experienced them. My sister explained that her son would sometimes run into her bedroom during the night, terrified and rambling. He had no recollection of having done so the following day, but my sister advised that these episodes often accompanied a cold or cough, as her son's often came when he had a temperature.

Christopher appeared to be well but unless signs of cold or viruses were obvious, we would not always be aware that he was feeling ill. In fact, when I actually thought about it, there was very little evidence that he was *ever* ill and in any event, the paediatrician did not mention that night terrors would be the result of ill health or a rise in temperature.

The episodes came infrequently during the months that followed and although we had grown accustomed to witnessing them, it was always distressing to see him awake from sleep so rapidly, looking terrified and not appearing to recognise where he was, or who we were.

Nevertheless, having been advised that night terrors were both common and harmless, we were not too concerned about Christopher's health until we received a message from the school one day informing us that he had collapsed shortly before being placed on the bus to return home. The school nurse advised that he had been walking around the classroom when he suddenly looked confused and had dropped swiftly to his knees. She described how he then stared ahead and was trembling slightly, as if shivering from cold.

Having witnessed many seizures herself, she was convinced that he had experienced an epileptic fit and when we rushed out to meet him off the bus a short while later he had a strange expression on his face. When our hands were held out to take his we were upset to see that he flinched away from us, as if frightened by the sudden movement. It was distressing to see him looking so scared but not wanting to make the situation any worse, we spoke softly to him and waited until he felt confident enough to walk with us.

We were now completely confused. The description of the episode which the school nurse had given sounded identical to the ones we ourselves had described to the paediatrician, with the exception that he had already been awake when it happened on this occasion and had not woken from sleep before the symptoms began.

The doctor was contacted, another referral was made for Christopher to be seen by the paediatrician and an appointment was arranged for just a few weeks later. During this next meeting we again described the episodes we had witnessed at home, before going on to describe the incident which had occurred at school, but we were surprised when the original diagnosis of night terrors was reaffirmed. It was true that we didn't understand much about them, but we were not convinced that it was possible to experience these *dream-like* states, without having fallen asleep in the first instance. Also, the school nurse had herself been convinced that she had witnessed an epileptic seizure and having to manage many other pupils with the same condition, we trusted her opinion.

The paediatrician left the room and re-entered with her colleague a few moments later, but having gone through the same description once again, her colleague agreed with the diagnosis. I was uneasy despite their insistence and after thanking the paediatrician for agreeing to meet Christopher, we left the hospital with the intention of making an appointment with the general practitioner.

The doctor listened to our concerns and was kind enough to make a referral to a neurologist at the same hospital, where the diagnosis of epilepsy was eventually given. I don't know why this particular diagnosis concerned me so much, but it did. I suppose up until this point Christopher had always appeared to be in good health and having seen how vulnerable and ill some of the other pupils were at school, I was again frightened about what the future would hold.

We were offered a prescription for epileptic drugs but we needed time to adjust to the news and to consider the pros and cons of administering such strong medication. Our biggest fear was that Christopher would suffer the side effect of liver damage to which we would feel completely accountable, if we decided to proceed with drugs.

I made another appointment with our doctor and he spoke to me about our concerns. Liver damage was a possibility, but it was low risk and if we began treatment and watched for any signs of jaundice, blood tests could be taken to ascertain if damage was being done. If this was found to be the case, treatment would immediately cease and serious damage could be avoided. If, on the other hand, we decided against treatment, there was a risk that Christopher would stop breathing because of the type of epilepsy which he experienced. Given the possible outcome of both scenarios I felt that there was very little choice.

The neurologist was contacted with our decision and Christopher was prescribed anti-convulsion drugs and for a few weeks all was well. There was no evidence of jaundice but his behaviour again began to deteriorate alarmingly, which had been another of the possible side-effects mentioned. We had been advised not to dwell on the list of side-effects, but to begin treatment with an open mind and we had done this. But with the severity of attacks at school escalating and this being mirrored in the behaviours presented back at home, he was taken off the medication within just a few months of starting it. An alternative medication was introduced with no noticeable behavioural disturbance and we were relieved to note that the increase in aggression which had erupted over the past few months slowly ebbed away.

The seizures continued and Christopher began to experience greater difficulties in breathing throughout the activity. Fortunately, each one typically lasted less than a minute, but he struggled to make 3 breaths in that time and his lips would turn blue. We were not too concerned by the ineffectiveness of the medication at this stage, as it was still being increased at regular intervals and the maximum dose had not yet been reached. However, as the weeks continued to pass and the seizures not only increased, but began to form a pattern, our anxieties grew.

Christopher would go approximately one month seizure-free, only to experience an average of 3 to 5 seizures within a 24 hour period. He was completed exhausted by the time he had had his third seizure and slept all day, with the exception of waking to have more. There was never any less than an hour between one seizure and the next and the maximum time between seizures would be 7 hours. We soon learned that the greater time elapsed between seizures, the fewer he would experience and on such occasions, he would often play in-between and be quite lively. However, if the time between seizures was less, then the more we could come to expect during the course of the day.

As Christopher was not being seen regularly by the neurologist or epilepsy nurse I devised charts on the computer to record the number, duration and description of seizures and on one particularly bad day, we were concerned to note that he had experienced a sixth. As he had been sleeping all day and was still completely exhausted we decided to contact the doctor for advice. We were not convinced that he would not have further attacks and as the pattern was different from what we had come to expect, we needed reassurance.

The doctor arrived shortly afterwards and asked for details of the seizures Christopher typically experienced. When he realised that they came in clusters, he was not concerned by the fact that he had never had as many as 6 in one day before. However, as Christopher did not awake during the examination which followed and we were still very concerned about what would happen if more seizures occurred, the doctor made arrangements for him to be seen at hospital where he was prescribed rectal diazepam.

The doctor advised us to use the diazepam in the event of any seizure lasting over a minute if there was no sign of recovery. We were also advised that if he recovered from one seizure but a further one followed within the space of fifteen minutes, it was to be treated as the same seizure and rectal diazepam was to be used. Further instruction was that *if* we were considering using diazepam, we should have already called the emergency services with a request for a paramedic to attend. This was in the event that rectal diazepam did not work and it would need to be given intravenously.

It was the first time that we realised that even *if* we knew how to administer mouth-to-mouth resuscitation on Christopher when he stopped breathing, it simply would not work. Apparently his chest muscles tightened during seizures which prevented the continuation of normal breathing. This was the reason that his lips turned blue over the course of the seizure and why he became so frightened beforehand. It had never been because of what he saw in his dreams it had been the realisation that he couldn't breathe.

This information must be difficult enough to deal with when the person understood what was happening to them. To someone with the understanding of a baby, it must be completely and utterly bewildering.

We left the hospital after Christopher had been examined once again. He lay against the back of his wheelchair completely exhausted, having lost another day to the epilepsy which would be with him throughout his life. The prescription for diazepam was handed in at the chemist and we received the same guidelines from the resident pharmacist. It would take up to five minutes to work and if we were considering using it, we should have already contacted the emergency services and requested that a paramedic attend.

The fact that we now had something constructive to do if Christopher did not recover from a seizure, gave us some reassurance. We did not want to dwell on the fact that if the diazepam proved to be ineffective, how long it was going to take for an ambulance to arrive at the door, or how long a person could last without oxygen before suffering further brain damage or even death.

. . . .

CHAPTER EIGHT

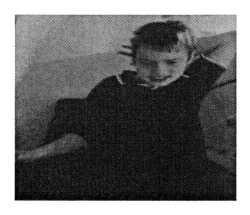

Christopher aged 12 years

As Christopher's epilepsy began to worsen it became apparent that his behaviour would deteriorate on the days leading up to seizures. It also became apparent that once the seizures had passed, his behaviour would once again settle. Of course, there were still occasions where he presented with challenging behaviour during seizure-free times, but the *probability* of behavioural deterioration around the time of seizures, was increased and it therefore became another recognised trigger.

Staff at school continued in their struggle to manage his behaviour on days when higher levels of aggression were being displayed and the decision was taken to cancel outings. Weekly activities such as shopping, swimming and horse riding were also stopped and day trips were no longer part of his school life.

This decision was taken because of the unpredictability of his behaviour, which had admittedly become quite erratic. The level of aggression charts which had been devised some years previously no longer gave an accurate account of the types of behaviours which could be expected in any given level, *or* of the time scale each level could last. Extreme level 3-type aggression could follow minutes or hours of calm as it had following his teeth extraction and would often take people by surprise. More often than not we could not locate any obvious trigger factors for such outbursts and were therefore unable to prevent them.

Christopher by now received 1-1 assistance in the classroom but additional staff were needed at many other times during the school day which meant that the teacher had to borrow colleagues from other classes. Two members of staff were always needed to assist at lunch-time and for the times when he was being moved from one place to another within the school, but the largest impact was for pad-changes. This task which had previously been completed by 2 members of staff would require as many as 6, during higher levels of aggression – one person to hold each limb, one to restrain Christopher's head so that he didn't bite and finally, one to carry out the actual task itself.

As there were many occasions when 1-1 support was not adequate a request had been made to the occupational therapist so that a specially adapted chair could be provided for use in the classroom. This did not affect the number of staff who was needed for pad-changes, but it did mean that activities and mealtimes would now only require one member of staff.

The chair was made from wood and looked typical in design, but it had been fixed onto a large wooden base on which Christopher could rest his feet. The base was only high enough off the ground to cater for the casters which were situated underneath and gave the chair its mobility. This meant that he could be moved around the classroom or school once seated. A 3-way harness prevented absconding and once seated a large wooden tray which acted as a table, slotted into place to complete the design.

We had completed home-school diaries since Christopher commenced his schooling and it was whilst we were reading through the teacher's comments for that day that we learned that the chair was also being used as a form of restraint when staff could not manage his behaviour. As we read further on, we were distressed to learn that he had not only been restrained in the chair for *that* entire school day, but also for the *previous* one.

At 9.00 o'clock the following morning Philip telephoned the head teacher to stress that we were unhappy for this to continue for 6 hours at a time, as Christopher was not able to occupy himself like a typical child could. His play ability still only consisted of sand, water and wheeled objects – none of which was offered to him whilst he was strapped into the chair, which must have left him bored as well as frustrated.

We understood the need for him to be removed from the other pupils when he was displaying aggression and asked if it was possible to find another solution to the problem, such as placing him outside in the enclosed play area or allowing him to access the school gymnasium, when the room was not in use.

If he was separated from other pupils using either of these options, it would solve the problem of him striking out at other children. Plus if the classroom assistant could observe him through the windows, they could ensure that he came to no harm without placing themselves at risk from attacks. The head teacher agreed to speak with the class teacher about our concerns to see if a compromise could be reached and assured us that he would let us know the outcome of any decisions.

Unfortunately, when we were contacted a short while later it was to inform us that our request was not considered to be feasible. The gymnasium was scheduled for frequent use by the individual classes throughout the week and when the weather was unseasonable, it would be impractical for Christopher to use the outside play area.

With no alternative solution being offered we were disappointed and concerned. If Christopher was unable to remain at school during times of aggression without him being restrained in a chair for this length of time, then we felt that we had no other option than to collect him. We advised the head teacher that if his behaviour deteriorated whilst he was at school, then we were to be contacted.

We suddenly realised that if he was displaying *any* signs of aggression in the morning there would be little point in sending him to school, as it would only result in a call to collect him a short while later. Having made the decision that we were to be contacted, we also realised that there would be occasions when we were not going to be at home, so to ensure that staff could contact us at any time during the school day we purchased our first mobile phone.

We had always understood that Christopher would not leave school at sixteen to attend college or begin work, as some of his more able peers would, but we had at least expected him to remain at school until he was nineteen years of age. Suddenly, we feared that this may no longer be the case.

The issue of schooling now looked very fragile but, despite the difficulties, the staff continued in their efforts to improve his ability to communicate and so with this in mind, we were invited to attend an informal meeting, along with two sets of other parents. The class teacher wished to demonstrate a new communication system she had recently discovered and we were interested to learn that video footage would be accompanying the demonstration.

As we sat with the other mums and dads we were advised that *all* of the children had made varying levels of progress and were thrilled to learn that this had been captured on video. It was so nice to learn of something positive for a change, especially as Christopher had not been singled out as the only child who had not progressed, but had seemingly been included with the other pupils.

The cassette was placed into the video recorder and we watched as the images showed the class teacher and one of the pupils sitting at opposite ends of a table. The teacher was holding a sweet between her finger and thumb and the child was being encouraged to pick up a card off the table and pass it to her in exchange for the sweet. Once the card had been handed over, the sweet was offered and the card replaced in its original place on the table. The teacher beamed as she advised everyone that we were seeing PECS carried out, which stood for Picture Exchange Communication System. We were completely stunned. This wasn't a new system at all, but the one we had asked that the school use with no success several years earlier. Even then, we had been told in the autism school that it had been well established in this country having been introduced from America years previously.

Whilst some of the other parents excitedly asked questions we sat in silence. However, as Christopher appeared on screen our frustration couldn't help but subside when we saw that he not only sat during *several* exchanges, but that he picked up the PEC card, unprompted, and offered it to the teacher. After the turmoil of the past few years it was a very emotional moment and I fought back the tears as I watched him repeat the procedure again and again.

He understood that he needed to offer the card in exchange of the sweet and I could find no words to describe my surprise and pride as he calmly completed the session. This was more progress than we could ever have wished for and we readily accepted the offered cards at the end of the demonstration, so that we could repeat the sessions at home.

In September 1999 the 2-hours of weekly respite we had received ceased, when Social Services failed to replace the two family aid workers who were leaving us. We were very sad to be saying goodbye to the workers who had supported our family for the past 1½ years and to those we now referred to as friends.

Although practical support ceased, we continued to receive some input from the social worker who maintained telephone contact with our family and attended school reviews. The community nurse also provided a friendly face during such times but annual reviews had by this time been replaced by 6-monthly ones.

At home we continued to struggle when Christopher's behaviour was at its height and new strategies were thought of for how to deal with contact tasks, such as pad-changing. Philip or I could complete pad-changes alone if he was displaying moderate levels of aggression, but during high levels of aggression we resorted to using a duvet. By wrapping this around Christopher's shoulders in a *cape-like* fashion so that it held his arms down at his sides, it prevented him from pulling us towards his mouth to bite. This then enabled pad-changes to be completed rapidly and with as little upset as was possible and was considered to be an appropriate method of restraint by the community nurse, given the extreme aggression which we sometimes faced.

Mealtimes were particularly dangerous and during such times he would typically be fed over the stable-door to prevent him from lunging towards the food, crockery or the person feeding him, whilst they held a plate and fork. Even so, his arm reach was substantial and face slapping, hair grabbing and thrown food were an inevitable outcome.

Baths were not an option when Christopher was very aggressive as the floor and the bottom of the bath were slippery through splashes and became too dangerous with him lunging forward to attack. Even so, he would climb the stairs and rattle the bathroom door to make his wishes known and protest when his request was refused.

He was very unstable on the stairs at the best of times but when his attention was focused elsewhere, in his haste to get where he was going, he would fall and stumble which angered him still further. We were often placed in dangerous situations but none compared to bringing him downstairs when his fury was at its height.

Attacks could be dangerous enough to deal with on flat surfaces, but being dragged, pulled, bitten, etc, on the minimal amount of space provided by each step, was absolutely terrifying, especially if the outburst occurred near the top.

However, as worrying as our having to deal with Christopher was in such a dangerous area of the house, there was no alternative. He could not be left to play and wander on steps when he was still unable to use them safely and on one occasion Michael had taken the lead and I was behind, struggling to hold onto the back of Christopher's clothing as he lunged frantically forward to attack his brother.

A duvet covered Michael's head and back so that he could help prevent his brother from falling downstairs without sustaining injuries himself and as I gripped the banister with my free hand to slow down our speed, I noticed that Christopher's feet were only making contact with the edges of each step. His head and body leaned at such an angle that he was almost horizontal and the only thing which was preventing his falling down the remainder of the stairway was Michael and my efforts at holding him back. As I recall how our own feet landed precariously during the commotion, I will never understand how we avoided serious injuries, but we sustained only bruising and cuts.

The feeling of guilt that Michael was being placed in this situation without any control was always at the back of our minds. We were the ones choosing to keep our youngest son at home and yet it affected family life as a whole. But Christopher was as much a part of our family as Michael and we loved our children equally. None of them were responsible for how things were and in a way we were all victims of circumstance.

On calmer days I looked into Christopher's eyes and saw the baby I had fallen instantly in love with. I hated the world at times, I hated our lives at times, but there was never a time when I hated my son. The overwhelming urge to protect him was always present along with a love so huge that it hurt. I just prayed that we would always have the strength and the ability to take care of him as he grew larger and stronger.

....

CHAPTER NINE

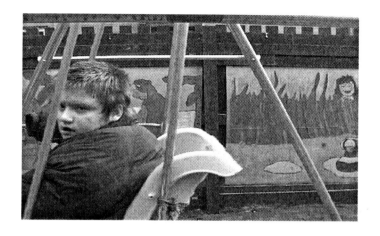

Christopher aged 13 years

It had been over a year since we had received any practical support from Social Services but the 2-hours of weekly respite was not particularly missed due to the conditions that had been attached. Sessions had been cancelled at frequent intervals as Christopher's behaviour remained unsettled, but although the actual ceasing of sessions did not in themselves have much affect, we found ourselves missing the contact that the support workers provided.

We were therefore pleased to be informed that 2 new support workers had been located to work with him and that we were being offered 3-hours of weekly respite. There were still conditions attached to us receiving this service and we were again requested to cancel sessions if he was displaying signs of aggression, but at least it was a step in the right direction.

As our own vehicle was larger than that of the support workers, we had also been asked if this could be used to transport Christopher and with our agreement, respite recommenced. Not having use of a vehicle during sessions did place restrictions on us but it was important for Christopher to be somewhere other than school or at home and so we accepted the inconvenience as inevitable.

There were occasions when he was returned home an hour or so earlier than scheduled without warning, and as this was a possibility, it meant that we were unable to leave the house or make plans for the time he was away, but we hoped that the situation would improve in the future.

In warmer weather he was taken for wheelchair rides around the boating lake a few miles away and during calmer sessions he typically enjoyed his visits there and often giggled as he was pushed around the scenic route. In wet weather a community centre which was used by other special needs children was sometimes available, although this had proven to be less of a success and Christopher sometimes remained in his buggy throughout the two hours the centre remained open, so that he could not attack the other children or harm himself.

His behaviour was remarked upon on several occasions, although it was true to say that he never attended sessions when he was displaying high levels of aggression and was always accompanied by his buggy.

However, whilst we accepted and recognised that the behaviours which were being displayed were *mild* in comparison to those which he *could* present with, to people with no knowledge of this, it came as a bit of a shock.

We explained that he could scratch or grab on most days and that as he had been diagnosed with *severe* challenging behaviour, it was unrealistic not to expect some milder behavioural problems. However, it was evidently not what the workers had anticipated and clearly not what they were used to.

At school, the head teacher had decided to create a class specifically for pupils with autism. Initially, he wanted to split the school day in two so that during the mornings, some of the affected children would attend a class together and in the afternoons they would rejoin their own class peers as usual. It was hoped that the proposed class would eventually continue throughout the day, but in the meantime we had been asked to contact the Director of Education in our own borough to support the proposal.

As children also attended the school from different boroughs, Directors from the various Educational Departments were also contacted by the head teacher in the hope of securing sufficient funding so that a teacher with experience in autism could be employed to head the group.

The proposal was successful and the class was now up and running, but although we had hoped that it would improve the situation if Christopher was separated into a smaller group along with children whose ability was more similar to his, it hadn't. Furthermore, since first joining the class some 11 weeks earlier, he had been excluded from school on 12 separate occasions.

In addition to these exclusions, he continued to remain at home if he was displaying any aggression in the mornings and if his behaviour deteriorated once he had actually arrived, we were contacted to collect him as agreed. There were occasions when we received calls within minutes of his arrival, but even when he remained at school for longer periods, he seldom made it to dinner time and was typically excluded by mid morning.

As the months passed by Christopher rarely completed a full week and we were further concerned to be given a letter from the escort which requested that we did not send him to school on a specific date *regardless* of his behaviour. The head teacher had taken the decision because there would be no male teachers present to assist the female staff should any difficulties arise and so, our biggest fear now regarded his future placement at the school which was looking particularly dismal.

The introduction of PECS which had initially looked so promising had been a short-lived success and problem behaviours often seriously impacted upon the sessions, sometimes making them impossible to complete. Christopher had no difficulty in understanding the basic principle of the system, i.e. that in order to be *given* something, he first had to *offer* something, but although he would offer a card he had not progressed to differentiating between the various pictures on them. In fairness, as he was still not displaying any interest in books, pictures or photographs I suspected that he was not yet ready to do so.

We had also noticed that when we were completing sessions at home, as the items which were being used for the exchanges were in view, things usually went smoothly. But as Christopher now associated *giving* something in return for *receiving* something, he would present any unfamiliar objects, in place of a card, throughout the day and immediately become distressed when we incorrectly guessed what it was he was asking for. As we continued to guess and offer unwanted objects, he then became increasingly angry and physically aggressive towards us. I suppose as far as he was concerned he was still offering a *ticket* and he did not understand why on one occasion he was being given something that he wanted, but on another occasion, he was not.

Medication reviews provided an opportunity to discuss problem behaviours with the psychiatrist, who had always felt that the majority of his aggressive outbursts resulted from his extensive communication difficulties and the inevitable frustration this caused. At one such review she asked what method of communication was being used and how long it had been in place. The class teacher provided the relevant details and although the psychiatrist stressed that she was a big advocate of PECS, she felt that it was too complex for Christopher to use given his ability. She advised that objects of reference would be easier for him to understand and with this advice more emphasis was placed on the latter means of communication.

We were disappointed that the system had not proven to be the success we had dreamed of, but with the mounting confusion it had caused during the past few months, we completely agreed with her opinion. Furthermore, as Christopher had instigated the use of objects many years earlier, it made sense that his own chosen means of communication was encouraged and given a fair chance, rather than being dismissed.

The continuing and repeated use of individual words over the years had also enabled Christopher to recognise a wider selection of *key words*. They were used in short or stinted sentences, but he now understood approximately 10 words. He displayed no interest in speaking, although it was apparent that he liked the sound of his own voice, as he often giggled loudly, screamed or '*sang*' in his own way.

The droning noise he made was quite melodious and we always passed positive comments when he *sang* and applauded him when he had finished. The praise always made him giggle as if he was extremely pleased with himself and it was lovely to see him wandering calmly around obviously gaining a great deal of pleasure from listening to the sound of his own voice.

There was still no improvement with the epilepsy and although 3 medications had now been used in an attempt to gain some control over it, Christopher continued to experience an average of 3 -5 seizures every 9 days or so. The rectal diazepam followed him around wherever he went, at school, at home and in a bag which we carried everywhere, just in case of emergencies.

The community nurse had arrived at our home one day with a suitcase on wheels and had joked about our being able to practice how to use the diazepam on a bottom. But, although we assumed that she was teasing, sure enough, when the case was opened up it revealed a model of the real thing. Even though it was plastic, I recall how my hands shook as I pulled the top off an empty container of diazepam and inserted its nozzle at a 45 degree angle. I was advised that Christopher's bottom would also need to be slightly elevated to avoid the liquid from leaking out once inside the rectum and that when the *real* container was empty, to squeeze his buttocks together before withdrawing the nozzle, so as to avoid the same. Although the experience had made me nervous, I understood how important it was for us to be able to administer the liquid in an emergency and hoped that even in a state of panic; instinct would take over now that I had completed the task on my own.

Since the demonstration, we had used the diazepam on several occasions, but only following a 5th seizure, to allow Christopher's body to have a rest. I had asked for advice and permission from the doctor to do so because the seizures were in clusters and, as the doctor felt that this was a good idea, permission had been granted.

He still typically experienced seizures whilst asleep, but over the past year there had been a noticeable increase in the amount of times he had been awake when activity occurred. The possibility of injuries occurring when he was awake was obviously far greater than if they happened when he was asleep, and so the stairs became an even greater hazard than they had been previously.

The garden steps were also a continuing concern and had proven to be a great inconvenience if he happened to be playing in the garden when he suffered a seizure. He was always shaky whilst in the recovery stage and unable to take his weight on his feet for 10 or so minutes afterwards, which resulted in the need for our carrying him up into the house. This was now almost an impossible task, but carrying him from one place to another was still a large part of our lives. There was little to choose between the weight of a thrashing fourteen year old, *or* the deadweight of Christopher following a seizure, but the latter was by far the most distressing to witness.

Our wait for a bungalow had continued and despite being regarded as a priority, the authority had no success in locating suitable property. The delay had been caused by a number of factors. The Council did not own any properties that were deemed to be suitable for Christopher and so the Director of Housing had decided to involve the services of a Housing Association so that one could be bought.

However, bungalows were well sought after in the borough and very few of them were actually situated entirely on the flat. Of the few which had been located many had steps either leading down to, or up from them, and some even contained steps inside to cater for the difference in the ground levels between lounges, hallways and kitchens. Also, whenever the Housing Association received brochures of bungalows that sounded as if they might be suitable, the occupational therapist had been unable to visit and assess them before they were sold, due to her excessive workload. The latter problem had been partly resolved when the Associations', Head of Housing, decided to view potential bungalows, accompanied by the report and specifications from the occupational therapist.

The idea being that *if*, having viewed a bungalow and it was still considered to be appropriate the occupational therapist would be contacted so that a professional assessment could take place. This would help prevent wasting time waiting for her to visit properties which were obviously unsuitable. If the property passed the assessment, we could then be contacted and allowed to visit. However, things had never progressed to this stage and we had never been invited to view any bungalows to date.

The wait was depressing and as dangerous as it had ever been and as Christopher now measured 5 feet 6 inches in height and weighed 10½ stone there were times we honestly believed that someone would be seriously injured or killed before we were actually re-housed. Having to carry him up and down concrete steps when he refused to walk was now a real nightmare and looking back to how we managed when he was just eight years of age, and struggling to do the same, made us realise how much easier that had been in comparison.

Home life was increasingly difficult but with the respite services once again deteriorating, we feared that things were about to get worse as sessions rarely passed by without comments or complaints. We had been invited to attend a meeting at the Department to discuss the main issue, which apparently regarded Christopher's ability to grab whilst harnessed in the back seat of the vehicle. We explained that the existing 3 point harness was not strong enough to prevent him from rocking forwards and despite the size of the vehicle; he could reach both the driver and front seat passenger when he had loosened the groin strap.

I also mentioned my concerns regarding the design of the current harness which had originally been issued. The harness had to be used in conjunction with a length of belt that remained in the vehicle at all times. The neck strap clicked into a fastener at the top end of the belt, but the belt had to be threaded in and out of the buckle-type fastener which was situated at the groin.

Whatever Christopher's mood type it was never wise to bend down in front of him as he was likely to tug hair, slap and scratch even in fun. Also, during higher levels of aggression it was *immensely* dangerous to get near the length of belt when he was kicking or lashing out, much less likely to complete a weaving-type action whilst warding off blows.

It was agreed that the present harness was not safe to use, but although a referral for a more appropriate one was made, we left the Department with as much anxiety as we had had on entering it. We knew from past experience that any harness would take several months to be approved and issued and in the meantime the problems surrounding his being able to reach and grab from the back seat of the car, would obviously continue.

Not only that, the issue relating to the harness might have been the *main* cause of concern, but it certainly was not the *only* cause. His behaviour in general was proving to be difficult to manage by the respite services and we had listened to endless accounts of incidents when Christopher had grabbed or scratched the support workers.

It was a frustrating situation. If Social Services were only happy to provide sessions when he did not display any problem behaviours – no matter how mild –

then the service would be virtually non-existent. As it was, sessions often ended early or were cancelled due to higher levels of aggression and although grabbing and scratching were not pleasant, and had always been actively discouraged, these types of behaviours did not pose any real threat to the workers safety.

As we made our way back home we wondered how long it would be before Social Services withdrew practical support altogether. We were a problem to the Education Department, a problem to the Housing Department and we had now become a problem to the Social Services Department.

CHAPTER TEN

....

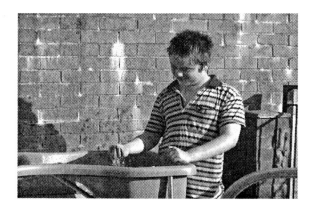

Christopher aged 14 years

As the issues regarding education and respite went from bad to worse, an acquaintance who knew about our circumstances asked if we had considered contacting an advocacy agency for advice. We explained that the conditions placed on Christopher receiving services, resulted from his challenging behaviour and not from him being disabled. And, as both the Education and Social Services Department had always maintained that it was appropriate to provide conditional services due to the risk factors involved, there seemed little point in doing so.

Over the following weeks however, we considered whether it might not be a good idea to seek an opinion from an independent agency and realised that we would have nothing to lose by contacting one for advice. If the authorities were within their rights to behave the way in which they currently were, then we would be no worse off. *If*, on the other hand, we *were* being treated unfairly, then the situation could only improve if we were armed with the facts.

We finally decided in favour of seeking outside assistance and a few days later an advocacy worker called on us at home. She discussed our difficulties at length and having decided to tackle the issue of education first, asked to examine Christopher's Statement of Educational Needs. We were bewildered when s*pecify* and *quantify* were mentioned with regards to the various therapies which he should have been receiving and so we asked for further explanations.

She advised that Christopher was entitled to receive therapies such as speech and language, hydrotherapy, etc, and that each therapy should be clearly named on the Statement. The Statement should also state how often the therapy was to be provided, how it was to be implemented, provide details of the duration and content of each session and finally state how many members of staff would be required to enable the therapy to be carried out. Apparently, *sufficient staff* was not a specific *or* adequate response.

The advocacy worker was also concerned that we were either being contacted to collect Christopher, or he was being restrained in a chair at school. She advised that if additional staff were needed for him to remain at school and to receive the same opportunities as the other pupils were, then the Education Department had a duty to provide funding for such.

We were baffled by this information and stressed that his behaviour could be particularly challenging, but were met with the same response. Additional assistance should be provided and the environment adapted to meet his needs, if necessary, to reduce risks, but his entitlement to receive education was the same as every other child.

Next we spoke about the issue of respite and were puzzled to receive much the same advice as before. The authority was under a clear duty to provide a service whenever a person had been assessed and recognised as meeting the necessary criteria. Services should not be rationed, non-existent or conditional on a *good behaviour* basis. We were advised to contact a solicitor who specialised in educational law to resolve the difficulties we were experiencing with school and informed that the issues of respite provision could also be dealt with by the same law firm.

Over the following weeks we found ourselves with a lot to mull over. The social worker had telephoned to advise that the Department was withdrawing respite services for health and safety reasons and the solicitor had confirmed that he was accepting our case against the education authority. The former issue was half expected and took a back seat whilst we collected any correspondence relating to Christopher's education, so that our case against the Department could be prepared and eventually submitted for tribunal.

In the meantime reviews continued at school, now every 3 months, and in addition to our own presence, were typically attended by the head and class teachers, community nurse and social worker. Reviews of his Statement of Educational Needs were obviously more important and in addition to the regular attendees, were the Special Education Needs Officer from our own borough, as well as a school representative from the borough in which the school was situated.

It was during one such review in July 2002 when we were accompanied by the advocacy worker, that we were completely astonished to hear the head teacher assure everyone present that he foresaw no further problems with future exclusions now that the autism morning class had been set up.

Typically quite an introverted person, but stunned by the ease in which the situation had been trivialised, I suddenly found myself stating that on *every* one of the 12 occasions in which Christopher had been excluded in the past 11 weeks, it was *during* the autism class in the mornings *and* not in the afternoon class as would have been expected. The embarrassing silence which followed was eventually broken by the head teacher's quiet admission that this was in fact the case, although he anticipated that things would settle in the future.

As the comments continued in a positive theme our astonishment grew. No one from the Education Department was going to take our concerns of a potential exclusion seriously, whilst the head of the school assured them that all was well. If it was a straight choice between believing a professional who should surely know what was happening in his own school, or concerns rambled by *anxious parents*, we had no hope of being taken seriously.

I felt completely and utterly let down. We had complied with *every* request that the staff had made. We had supported the school in securing 1-1 assistance and we had supported them in securing a teacher experienced in autism. But instead of them being honest with the Education Department about their inability to properly support Christopher's complex needs, they painted an entirely different picture of what was actually happening.

I thought of his home/school diary and the endless comments regarding concerns about escalating behaviour. I thought of his decreasing attendance due to the number of aggressive days we were experiencing. I thought of the days when we were contacted to collect him, days when the school simply would not allow him to attend – regardless of his behaviour – and I thought of the mobile phone which we had carried around like an additional body part since 1999. ...And finally I thought of the activities his class peers were able to enjoy whilst he remained in the classroom each day, sometimes restrained and miserable.

As the meeting ended we made our way home, tired and frustrated. If the teachers had stressed their concerns to the Education Department, then additional support might have been provided. As it was, no help would be forthcoming because, as far as the Department was concerned, it simply was not needed. It had been a wasted opportunity and the beginning of a breakdown in communication between us and the staff at school.

The following 3 days Christopher attended school and remained there throughout each day. However, his behaviour deteriorated in the afternoons and we were not surprised to be contacted to request that we collect him in our own vehicle, as there were concerns about placing him on the school bus. This was for the 9th, 10th and 11th of July 2002.

With the summer holiday nearly upon us we were almost relieved. At least we knew that there would be no complaints and exclusions during this time, as Christopher would be at home. The break would also provide us with the opportunity to de-stress and let our recent anger with the school subside before the beginning of the autumn term.

During the summer break we still managed to complete trips on calmer days, using the same methods that we had used during subsequent years – arriving early at destinations and leaving before the crowds descended. Admittedly, there were some places we could no longer visit and some activities which we could no longer do, but on the whole we tried to remain positive and integrate as best as possible.

The canal boat rides which we had enjoyed since Christopher had been a baby were no longer attempted, as we could not safely restrain him when he was being taken out from his buggy to transfer him to the boat. In fairness, even if this could have been accomplished, as he would then have to have been harnessed throughout the 3-4 hours trip – to prevent him from hanging over the boat's side trying to play with the water – it would not have been much fun for him.

It was a shame in some respects because in every other way it had been a perfect choice for a day out. The gentle humming of the boat and constant movement had proven to have a relaxing quality about it and the wildlife along the canal bank, as well as in the canal itself, was both stunning and interesting to observe.

But although the choice of destinations had decreased somewhat, over the past few summers we had been fortunate to have had use of some fields through Philip's past employer and friend, who rented a farm some 6 miles from our home. Different fields became available once cows were moved to new ones and if the weather was nice, we would pack a hamper and go for picnics. Once the gates were closed behind us, Christopher could wander around in perfect safety and this enabled us to relax for a couple of hours and forget about what was happening back at home.

Sometimes he would take our hands and enjoy walking around the perimeter of the fields, and on other occasions he simply enjoyed running freely with the breeze brushing against his face and hair. During the times when he was particularly hyperactive being able to run around for several hours was so therapeutic, as was it when he was distressed or anxious and he would return home much calmer than he had been on leaving it.

The farm also provided him with the opportunity to see animals at close range and whenever Philip's friend asked if we could help with the cows, we were always happy to oblige. Whilst Philip milked the cows in the diary, Christopher would be wheeled into the barn to watch as I made sure the calves had enough milk, cake and hay to last overnight.

When he was particularly calm it was lovely to see him touching the calves and he thoroughly enjoyed being nuzzled by the resident farm dog, Meg, who seemed to sense that he had problems. It was funny how perceptive animals could be as we noted how our own two cats tolerated much more fussing or contact from him, than they would from anyone else.

The summer holiday passed by rapidly and despite problem behaviours during the months which had led up to the long break, we had only had two difficult days in the whole of the 6 weeks. We were relieved and felt better than we had in a long time, and we hoped that the return of the school routine would be coped with just as well.

The first few days passed without any significant problems but it was soon apparent that Christopher really did not wish to return to school. His behaviour deteriorated as soon as he was being washed and dressed in the mornings and when we managed to carry him to the bus, we typically had to place him in the harness ourselves as the escorts could not manage to do so.

Once there, he would typically protest in the only way he knew how, which was to attack those around him and we were then contacted to collect him. It was a vicious circle and although we felt that it was important to have attempted to see if he would settle, with the increase in calls requesting that he be returned home, we again began to cancel school on the days when he was displaying aggression.

By this time the solicitor was in contact with both the Education Department and the school itself, to see what efforts were being made which would allow Christopher to return, and remain at school, during times of high levels of aggression. It was felt that staff could manage him if he was away from the other pupils, but without any spare classrooms available, this would not be possible.

We were invited to attend a further meeting along with the social worker and community nurse where it was suggested that if Christopher's school day was reduced to just 2 hours, he could return to school, with the same conditions that were in place before. Those being, that he did not attend school if he was aggressive in the mornings and we would have to collect him if his behaviour deteriorated once there.

The social worker and community nurse seemed satisfied with this plan, but we simply could not believe what was being offered. As Christopher's behaviour had been, at best, unpredictable for the past few years and that it was almost consistently *bad* at school, he would be absent or returned home on a daily basis. The only thing that would actually alter was that instead of 6 hours of schooling being provided with unsatisfactory conditions, he was now being offered just 2.

We sat in silence for a few moments to digest what had been said. The head teacher evidently wanted us to make a decision there and then but as the solicitor was already in the process of preparing our case for tribunal, we stated that we did not feel that we were in a position to decide one way or the other without first seeking advice. With the matter left undecided, there seemed little point in continuing with any potential plans regarding where Christopher would spend the 2-hours at school and what he would do during that time, if the offer was accepted. True, the 2-hours was only to be provided on a temporary basis, as it was hoped that if he was manageable this could be increased over time. But then considering his current behaviour, how likely was it that he would suddenly improve in any event, and how long exactly was a *temporary* basis?

On the journey home Philip and I discussed our feelings in greater depth. What I found difficult to understand was the reasoning behind the offer. The Education Authority was already aware of our dissatisfaction with the conditions placed on Christopher attending school, since we had been in possession of the full facts. …And yet, they were now intending to place additional conditions – on top of those which we were already dissatisfied with.

When we arrived home a short time later Philip contacted the solicitor to inform him of the latest developments and to our relief we were advised to refuse this offer. Christopher had the right to attend unconditional schooling and if additional staff or adaptations to the environment were required for this to happen, then the Education Authority was under a duty to ensure that it did.

Following our refusal to accept the offered two hours of schooling each day and request that the standard 6-hours be provided instead, we received a letter from the school stating that without agreeing to the conditions, Christopher would be unable to return as a pupil. Although the term had not been included in the letter, he had, in effect, been permanently excluded.

. . . .

CHAPTER ELEVEN

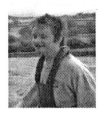

Christopher in 2003

As the weeks passed by we continued to care for Christopher at home without any outside support or practical assistance. All of the outside chores, such as food/clothes shopping, paying bills, etc, were left for Philip to complete whilst I remained at home to look after Christopher.

The solicitor had arranged for a psychologist to visit so that an assessment could be made and a report had now been completed, which was to be included with the bundle for tribunal. Although the report, primarily dealt with the issue of education, we noted that it also contained comments regarding the lack of support we were receiving from Social Services. The sentence which immediately stood out from the rest being, *exceptional difficulties, in the writer's opinion, should have resulted in an exceptional response and not a response that effectively says, Christopher's case is too complex for Social Services to support.*

With the Department reinstating respite services that very month, we joked that a copy must have been sent to the social worker instead of the solicitor, but the opinion was interesting as it concurred with the information we had been given by the advocacy services the previous year.

On this occasion we had been offered 2-hours of respite every 2nd to 3rd week, which was irregular but at least it meant that we were again headed in the right direction. The support workers took Christopher for drives and we had been asked if our vehicle could once again be used for this purpose, and of course, the same conditions had been attached as they had always been.

The referral for the harness which had been made several months earlier had not resulted in its arrival. The implementation of drives had also therefore seemed to be a strange choice of respite provision, given that the main risk factor involved in deciding its withdrawal last time, had regarded safety when travelling and the inappropriateness of the current harness. Nevertheless, we had accepted the conditions for the present time, with the knowledge that we would be pursuing this issue once the matter of schooling had been resolved.

Since his exclusion the education authority had placed a great deal of effort into locating and securing a placement in another special needs school and even though our main concerns centred on our son, I could sympathise with their dilemma. Having been assured staff were in control of the situation and they could foresee no more problems with future exclusions, the decision to do just that some 12 weeks into the new term, must then have come as a complete shock.

There were already plans to build a unit in the school and the Special Education Needs Officer was hopeful that it might be used for Christopher. The unit would be completed by the end of September 2003 and would have its own splash area, soft play area, changing facilities and also its own outside play area. It sounded perfect and having informed the solicitor that we were satisfied with the progress being made, the tribunal was cancelled and the bundle placed in safe keeping for future reference.

It was recognised that integrating Christopher with other children had not worked in the past and so a teacher with experience of autism had been employed to teach him separately. A classroom assistant was also employed to provide 2-1 support and, as the unit would not be ready for some months, a temporary venue had to be located in the borough.

A community centre for special needs children was considered to be a viable option as one of the rooms, which was to later accommodate a hydrotherapy pool, was not currently being used. We were invited along to the proposed venue to meet with a teacher and teaching assistant and having been shown the room, which had access to its own enclosed play area, we began the process of getting to know each other.

The teacher followed Christopher around and asked many questions regarding his abilities, likes, dislikes, etc, and it soon become apparent that she had not been given any information about him. Having realised this I offered to provide photo-copies of past statements so that she could see what stage of development he was at and what he was able to do.

The meeting went well and with the room being accepted, we agreed to Christopher initially receiving a reduced school day of 4-hours and also to transporting him to and from the venue ourselves. The centre had no facilities for providing hot meals and so we also agreed to bring a packed lunch, but at least he would be receiving some kind of education and with the proposed plans for 2-1 support in the special needs school, the situation finally looked much brighter.

Christopher settled into the new routine remarkably well, although after just four days the teaching assistant decided to leave the post and seek alternative employment. Her hasty departure meant that a temporary assistant had to be located until the vacancy was filled, but the teacher ploughed along undeterred by the hiccup. Within days the Education Department had managed to find a new assistant to fill the position and it was lovely to note how much Christopher looked forward to going to school each day. The placement evidently suited him and not sharing the room with other children lessened his anxiety, which in turn, lessened the aggressive outbursts which had admittedly become substantial during the past few years of schooling.

Of course, other children used the centre and a large room which was situated in the middle of the building was used as a playgroup. The upper half of the room was mainly made up of windows which enabled the light to penetrate through and provided an ideal place to display various pieces of art-work which had been produced during the session.

As the centre was used as an opportunities group, various activities were also going on throughout the day for older children and young adults to enjoy. We knew that keep fit classes were held during the week and that the centre was always busy with activity, but apart from being aware that the opportunities being offered were aimed at individuals with special needs, we knew very little else about the centre.

The weeks seemed to fly by and as the Easter Holidays approached we received news that funding had finally been secured to buy and install the hydrotherapy pool. This was fantastic news for the centre, but meant that another venue needed to be located following the holidays, as the placement in the school was not ready. This was a huge blow to the Education Department who had already thoroughly searched the borough before identifying this placement. It also meant that having settled into one venue, Christopher would now have to settle into another, before finally being moved on for the third, and hopefully, last time.

Being moved around so much in such a short space of time made us feel very anxious about how well he was going to cope. We were also anxious about whether the Education Department would be able to locate another venue in the minimal amount of notice they had been given, as failing to do so would result in Christopher remaining at home again, possibly for some time.

The Special Education officer was faced with a real challenge but again placed enormous efforts in attempting to locate another temporary venue in which schooling could take place. She drove around the borough considering any building which might be appropriate and days later we were asked to view a community hall.

The hall was in a quiet location with easy access for wheelchair and parking, but had no suitable outside play area. As Christopher loved to be out in the fresh air we felt that this could prove to be a problem, as the hall was quite small and much of the space was already taken up by the resident tables and chairs. An outside play area would therefore be important and would allow him to have his own space, if needed, which was something that would not be possible in just one room.

As the search continued we offered assistance and whenever we went for drives in the car we were constantly looking for suitable venues. Family also joined in and soon we were all throwing ideas around, but it was finally the Education Officer, who once again managed to locate a venue. She had apparently been driving along when she happened upon a small church which was situated in its own grounds. I recall how I laughed when she said that she had glanced skywards just moments previously and had desperately asked for divine intervention when she suddenly saw a notice board which was standing in the grass.

Having parked the car, she wrote the caretaker's details down and telephoned to see if the attached church hall was available. The church was just moments away from our own home, situated on the main road which we pass on a daily basis, but we had never really noticed it before. And yet, as we stood on the pavement outside, we agreed that it was absolutely perfect. It looked like one building from the outside, but it had been separated into three sections which were independent of each other. The church was situated in the front of the building and a hall was situated at the back. The middle section of the building - which was a good size, but much smaller than the other two - was used as a storage room, and this could be accessed from both the hall at the back and church at the front.

The hall was a lovely size and contained its own bathroom and well equipped kitchen and both were beautifully decorated and well maintained. The grounds around the building were again, a lovely size and entirely made up of a well kept lawn. And finally, a fence and secure gate completed the criteria. It was ideal. We could park directly outside, walk Christopher the few paces from the pavement to the gate, and he would be perfectly safe. It was quiet and with the warm weather already upon us, the grassy play area would be well utilised and thoroughly enjoyed.

With the added bonus of a microwave, we now could cook him a hot meal at home which could later be re-heated. He always preferred eating a hot meal to having sandwiches and although we ensured he came home to a cooked tea, we knew that he had missed his midday school dinner.

The teacher and teaching assistant was as impressed as we were. They had struggled for the past 3 months without support or proper facilities and use of a kitchen meant that they could now enjoy hot refreshments at some point during the day. A bathroom in such close proximity also meant that one person was only left alone to supervise Christopher for a minimal amount of time and put less pressure on them during toilet breaks.

The venue was accepted and we were once again delighted to note how well he adapted to this new environment and settled without any significant difficulties. Of course days were still occasionally lost through high levels of aggression and also from the worsening epilepsy and during a review the education Department asked that we attend a hospital in Birmingham.

Although the suggested doctor specialised in the treatment of epilepsy, as there was behavioural deterioration prior to seizures, the Department hoped that if seizure control could be accomplished, behaviours would improve. We agreed to the referral as we had already stressed our concerns that Christopher was not seeing any specialist on a regular basis. However, we reminded the Department that he had only experienced seizures since he was eleven, but had presented with severe challenging behaviour all of his life and would continue to do so, with or without full seizure control.

Nevertheless, the appointment was scheduled for just a few weeks time and we visited as agreed. The visit itself was not quite what we had anticipated and the doctor seemed confused that we had travelled to the hospital at all. She stressed that she had great confidence in Welsh doctors and felt that she had little else to contribute to what had already been achieved.

However, the doctor was interested by the severe aggression which Christopher could present with and stated that in terms of the severity and duration of attacks, he was only one of six disabled people in Britain whose behaviour was so severely affected. The level 3-type behaviours we described were of equal interest to her and once we stated that Christopher only presented with this level of aggression following sleep, she felt that this was a case book type of seizure. The confusion was now spreading as we could not understand how anyone could be wide awake, fully focussed on their surroundings, the people around them and yet attack with such ferocity whilst in the grip of a seizure. It made no sense to us and was certainly unlike any of the seizures Christopher was known to have, but the doctor seemed convinced.

As the appointment drew to a close the doctor informed us that she would contact the general practitioner and psychiatrist to recommend that a specific medication be prescribed for use during the level 3-type behaviours. She explained that if she was correct and that a seizure was in process, his behaviour would respond to the medication. We thanked her and left for the long journey home.

Philip contacted the Education Department the following day to let them know how the appointment had gone. They seemed disappointed that a miracle cure was not going to be forthcoming and that the proposed medication would not have any positive impact upon staff's management of Christopher on a daily basis. We were then asked if we would be prepared to allow him to undergo a 12-week epilepsy assessment in a specialist unit in Cheshire. This request was completely unexpected and when we realised that we would not be permitted to stay at the unit with him, we were full of apprehension and greatly distressed.

Our concerns about his worsening condition left us unable to refuse the offer, whilst our anxiety about leaving him alone, without him knowing why we were doing so, left us wishing that we could. But people die each year from poor seizure control and each time he experienced a seizure he fought to breathe. The choice was a difficult one to make, but we agreed.

A few weeks later we received information from the unit which described what the assessment would entail and gave details of the on-site school, residential buildings and occupational facilities. It appeared that most of the assessments were carried out on individuals with varying degrees of disabilities and that the on-site houses mentioned, accommodated and catered for approximately 6 children during their stay. Several staff members had responsibility of the children, some of whom needed 1-1 support and adults undergoing assessments were catered for in a similar way.

The letter explained that before any plans could be made for an assessment Christopher would first need to visit the unit. We were given a date to attend and advised that on arrival we were to go to a specific house with Christopher, who would remain there with staff whilst Philip and I were shown around the school, unit and other facilities. Dinner would be provided for us in the school canteen and the tour would continue afterwards, ending at around 5.00pm

When the day finally arrived we left the house in the early hours of the morning to keep our 9.00 appointment. We were armed with enough pads, bottles, refreshments and changes of clothing to last the day and hoped that the roads would be as kind to us as they had been when we visited Birmingham weeks earlier. The journey was long and as the warmth of the sun became stronger it was uncomfortable and sticky inside the car, but we were fortunate not to have been delayed in traffic for significant periods of time and Christopher remained in good spirits.

When we came to the final turning on the map we found ourselves entering, what was in effect a village-type community. The houses, unit, hospital, etc, were all contained within its substantial grounds and situated back from the main road. It was impressive, a little intimidating and certainly not what we had expected. We noticed that the houses had been given names such as elm, oak, ash, etc, and having registered our arrival in the reception area of one building, we made our way to the house name which had been listed on the letter we had received. We were warmly greeted and having freshened Christopher up in the bathroom, we awaited the arrival of the doctor who was to escort us around the unit.

Christopher had been excellent throughout the drive, but having been un-strapped from his buggy he became a little agitated in the room and so we asked if we could take him out into the garden. When the doctor finally arrived we realised that the plans which had been detailed in the letter, were not going to materialise. Instead of being shown the unit, we were asked if one parent could remain with him whilst the other one answered questions inside the house.

The process of answering further questions by different members of the team was repeated at intervals throughout the day and whilst Philip continued to supervise Christopher, I was summoned to the same room each time. Lunch was provided by the staff that brought a large tray into the garden and despite the slight drizzle in the air, we remained outside until it was time for us to make the return journey home.

We were exhausted and relieved when we finally boarded the car but wondered why the planned scheduled had been sent to us, only to be ignored. Still, in our anxiety to get back to our own home we soon put our confusion to the back of our minds. I glanced at Christopher who had been so good given the circumstances and prayed that things would work out for the best. I could not imagine leaving him in a strange environment with people he did not know and as I considered his confusion and distress at us doing this, I found silent tears rolling down my cheeks. He would be completely and utterly distraught and yet the doctors only looked at him in terms of his age and condition – not as the baby he was, albeit, in a young man's body.

During the next few days I tried not to dwell on the assessment, or on how Christopher would cope at being left. I knew it would be for the best if it meant that the seizures would be controlled and we didn't have to watch helplessly, as he fought to breathe and failed.

When the letter finally arrived I let Philip open it and prepared myself for the worst. Twelve weeks was a huge amount of time and in some ways, we would find it just as difficult to be without Christopher, because we knew how distressed he would be without us.

As I waited for Philip to speak I suddenly realised that he was offering the letter to me. He looked confused more than anxious and I wondered what was wrong. I took the piece of paper and forced myself to concentrate on its contents. The doctors apologised for not being able to offer Christopher an assessment but advised that they did not have the right type of facilities to cater for his needs. I didn't know how to react or whether I was to feel relieved or annoyed. The information we had previously received boasted exceptional facilities for disabled individuals, many of whom had challenging behaviour – there had been no mention of possible exclusion due to higher or more complex needs and yet this is exactly what had been done.

....

CHAPTER TWELVE

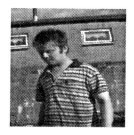

Christopher aged fifteen years

It had been four months since respite had been re-instated but although it had not been necessary to cancel sessions because of problem behaviours, we had regularly needed to do so because of seizures. We therefore made the decision to ask that respite be placed on hold until such time as it would benefit Christopher. There seemed little point in doing anything else when we were forever telephoning to say that he was *sleeping*, having had seizures the night before, or *sleeping* because he had been having seizures that day.

Schooling in the church hall had continued to go well and with just a few weeks left before Christopher was due to start the new special school, we were invited to view the room which he was now to have. The unit which had originally been suggested was now going to be used by some of the existing pupils instead and arrangements had been made for their old room to be adapted for Christopher's use.

As the unit had already been planned prior to his exclusion, and he was not yet a pupil, I felt that this was a fairer decision, but one that would affect what we had originally been offered and accepted, nonetheless. The changing facilities, soft play area and the splash area had all been designed specifically for the unit and this meant that Christopher would not have access to any of these. As he would remain in the classroom throughout the day and not be included in outings, swimming, horse-riding, etc, the splash area would have been a great asset, as it was one of the few activities he actually enjoyed and so we were admittedly a little disappointed.

As I looked around the room I tried to be positive. It was a good size and as it had been stripped of most of its furnishings, Christopher would have enough space to wander around without bumping into things. A single table and a couple of chairs was all that remained and these had been positioned in the corner of the room, to be used for various activities and also during lunch times. The carpet was being replaced with a type of cushion-floor which was both practical and smart and, most importantly, he would not be sharing the space with 6 or 7 other children.

On our immediate right there was a type of recess in which a large vinyl-covered mattress had been laid. This provided a quiet space in which he could withdraw to if things became too much for him to cope with. On our left was a door which led into another slightly smaller room and we were advised by the deputy head teacher that both rooms were included in the placement. A third door opened into a large cupboard and it was hoped that this could later be adapted and equipped to enable pad-changes to be completed. This would then eliminate the risk of Christopher harming other pupils whilst he walked through the school to the existing changing facilities.

As the flooring was still being fitted we were unable to pass through the fourth and final door which led to the play area. A single pathway ran from this play area and ended at the perimeter fence, where a gate had been fitted. This would enable us to enter the school whilst avoiding the busy main reception area. Everything seemed to have been considered and in all honesty, if we hadn't initially been told about the different facilities that would have been available, we would have been delighted with what was now being offered.

Although it looked bare in comparison to typical classrooms, we did not feel that this was necessarily a bad thing. Though, we were a little concerned at how Christopher was going to be kept occupied throughout the day if he was not able to leave the room and there were no facilities or equipment there for him to use. We hoped that this was because the rooms were not yet finished as we prepared to end the visit.

As we left the school we were assured that the placement would be completed by the end of September as anticipated. Christopher would initially receive a reduced school day of 4 hours 15 minutes Mondays - Thursdays and 4 hours on Fridays. We would be responsible for transport in the short term, but it was hoped that if he settled in well the school day could be increased and transport would then be included in the package.

If the issue of schooling was suddenly looking brighter, then so was the issue of accommodation and having continuingly failed to locate a suitable bungalow it was felt that one would need to be purpose-built. We had had several meetings during the past few months and with the involvement of an architect and surveyor, plans had already been drawn up and submitted to the Welsh Assembly for approval.

The project was to be a 3-way venture and involved the Council selling a piece of land to the Housing Association, on which they would build the property and so, become our new landlords. The property could only ever be rented throughout Christopher's life, after which time, it would be used to benefit another family with similar needs. But before the project could get underway, permission had to first come from the powers that be.

We realised that there was a very fine line to be drawn when it came to stressing the difficulties which we experienced. If *too* little emphasis was placed on our problems, then the Assembly might feel that a purpose-built bungalow would not be necessary. However, if the occupational therapist's report was *too* alarming, then it might be felt that it would be preferable to place Christopher in care, for our safety. In either one of those events, the bungalow would be refused.

Having seen the architectural drawings, we suddenly became pessimistic of the outcome. The building looked enormous and although the accompanying report was detailed and comprehensive, we were convinced that the Welsh Assembly would either reject the project out-of-hand, or demand that the architect dramatically downscale. However, with the necessary information having been submitted, there was nothing else to do, but wait.

Although we were concerned about the decision, this took a back seat when Christopher's seizures began to alter. As I comforted him during one such episode, I was alarmed to notice his head making backward jerking-type movements. This had never occurred before and as it was accompanied by high-pitched noises – similar to frightened screams and grunts - we contacted the neurologist for advice.

The neurologist was unconcerned by the alteration and stressed that it was quite normal for seizure symptoms to alter over time, but as the medication had had no effect on the number of seizures which Christopher was experiencing, she decided the time had come to prescribe a different medication. She stressed that it was unlikely that full seizure control would ever be possible and proceeded to advise of the potential side-effects of the drug she was about to prescribe.

We were given various dates to decrease and finally withdraw the present medication, whilst introducing and increasing the new anti-convulsion drug until it reached optimum dosage. Over the years we had become accustomed to doing this and on some occasions it had been necessary to juggle the management of 4 separate medications, whilst increases and decreases were made to specific ones, on specific dates.

We were not concerned about our ability to do this, but having now tried several drugs which had had no effect, we were concerned that Christopher would eventually experience seizures daily. Since they had first begun, the days between seizures had continually decreased and having seen the horrendous affects on families' unfortunate enough for this to happen, we were scared of what lay ahead.

However, 6 days later, and still only administering the introduction dosage, there was no sign of activity. 2 weeks later, the situation remained the same and by the end of the month there was still no sign of seizure activity. By the end of the following month, Christopher remained seizure-free and we wondered if the drug would continue to work. None of the previous medications had worked, even for the briefest amount of time and yet even at its lowest introductory dose, it had prevented activity from occurring.

There finally appeared to have been a breakthrough and with the additional news that the bungalow had been given the *green light* we were ecstatic if somewhat stunned. The Assembly had passed the *entire* project, without conditions or compromises and the surveyor had contacted us to advise that planning permission could now be applied for.

Unfortunately, this is when the problems really begun. The site had been owned by the Housing Department since 1957 and although it had been ignored for decades, this year it had been used as the venue for the local festival. It was large enough to accommodate both and as the festival only took place every 2nd year, we asked if it could be shared. But a local Councillor refused the suggestion and requested that the land be transferred from the Housing

Department to the Recreational Department instead. Months later, and despite planning permission being passed, the request resulted in the Council renegade on its previous decision to sell the land to the Housing Association.

The decision came as a huge blow, as following the Council's initial agreement to sell the land it had been tested and surveyed at a substantial cost to the Housing Association. The plans which had been submitted and passed by the Welsh Assembly Government had given details of the site and now we were in a position where permission had been granted to build the bungalow, but there was no place to build it.

In desperation, we contacted a solicitor who gave the Council a 20-week deadline to locate an alternative site. Searches had already been made throughout the borough but to date the land located had either been too small, or was owned by Parke Estate, coal-board or private. We were in regular contact with the regeneration officer and invited her along whilst we drove around the borough, searching for possible plots and although many were noted, none later proved to be viable.

To be so close and yet so far away from securing a safe home for Christopher and ourselves, after so many years of struggling, was distressing beyond words and yet we fought on. If a site was finally located we didn't know if the plans would need to be re-submitted to the Assembly and even if this was not the case, planning permission would still have to be sought once again, putting us months behind schedule.

With only a few weeks remaining before the solicitor was to take action, the Chief Executive of the Council telephoned to inform that a site had been located. He gave Philip directions to a road in a nearby village and asked that he meet him there for his opinion. As I waited at home with Christopher I prayed that it would be suitable and that things could once again start moving, but I was apprehensive. Things never tended to run smoothly and as I looked around the home we had shared for the past fifteen years, I realised that I could never imagine leaving it. Perhaps we were never intended to do so, I didn't know, but I simply could not imagine moving from here to the bungalow which had been designed for Christopher.

Half an hour later and Philip had already returned home to collect us. We boarded the car and drove a short distance in silence, before he turned away from the main road and drove down, what could easily have been mistaken to be a small country lane. I glanced across at him, confused by the unfamiliar surroundings, wondering where he was taking us and if he had taken a wrong turn, when he suddenly pulled up alongside an overgrown patch of land on our left and asked me what I thought.

For a moment I remained confused. I was expecting to see a piece of flattened land at the end of the journey but instead, found myself looking at a mass of trees, brambles and rubble. Then my eyes focused on the 20 foot high stone wall which acted as a backdrop to the area and I realised that this was being offered as a site on which to build the bungalow.

The land was directly below the village's main road and although the upper part of the wall was visible from the road above, it looked just like any other average wall. What was not visible or apparent from the main road, was that the wall continued down behind the huge drop, starting from the site upwards.

As I looked around I noticed that there were no other houses in close proximity. The wall was on the left of the road and a river ran on the right. There were a few houses scattered opposite and a single house further up the road, but the site was mainly surrounded by trees and a then, woodland. I realised that with so few homes in the vicinity, there would be far less noise to aggravate Christopher's intolerance and equally as important, he would not upset or annoy neighbours either when he was screaming, or *singing* loudly.

A more suitable piece of land could never have come our way. The amenities were situated on the main road above and if that wasn't convenient enough, the local surgery was just a 5 minutes walk. The thought of having to register with new doctors had been a real concern as we were fortunate to have some of the best in the borough and so, our decision was immediate. Philip contacted the Chief Executive directly from the site to confirm that we were delighted to accept it and arrangements were made for planning permission to be submitted.   With the news that it would not be necessary to contact the Assembly again, as it was simply a matter of transferring the bungalow from one site to the other, our relief was complete.

A few weeks later planning permission had been granted and the process of clearing the site had begun. The bungalow was expected to be completed within just 26 weeks time, which meant that we should be moving home sometime in September 2004. The fight to secure a suitable site had meant that we were a year behind schedule, but we no longer cared. We could finally say goodbye to the home which held so many bad memories for us and look forward to a new beginning.

CHAPTER THIRTEEN

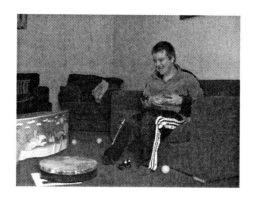

Christopher aged 16 years

Christopher had been in his new placement for almost a year and things were going surprising well. He continued to enjoy schooling and happily walked to and from the car on most days. He also now willingly walked along the pathway and into the classroom and so, it had not been necessary to resort to using the buggy.

He coped far better in his new environment as even though he was now being taught in a school, he did not have much contact with other pupils. Some of the other children would approach the fence of his play area to talk to him and although he could not speak, he mostly tolerated the interest from a distance and sometimes responded with smiles.

It was lovely to learn that some of the pupils made the effort to communicate with him even though they knew he could not vocalise his thoughts and it struck me how much empathy and understanding these children had, despite the fact that they had moderate to severe learning difficulties themselves. Another way, in which they often surpassed their more-able counterparts, is by recognising that Christopher sometimes responded negatively to attempts to communicate with him, but it was not meant to be personal. They recognised that his mood and behaviour regularly altered and simply accepted it without question.

Within a few months of him becoming a pupil at the school the head teacher had asked to see us in her office and although Christopher's home-school diary had shown little reason for us to be concerned, past experience left us with a feeling of foreboding. However, the head teacher had wished to speak to us about another child. She explained that the potential pupil had also been diagnosed with autism, was a year younger than Christopher and she asked if we had any objections to him using the second room of the 2-roomed placement until the end of term.

We had been relieved not to have been summoned to discuss problems about behaviours and totally confused that we had been asked permission from the head teacher to use a classroom in her school. The head teacher had assured us that the two boys would have little contact with each other, as the other boy could integrate with the other pupils more and join other classes at various points throughout the day. We had obviously agreed to the suggestion and left the school a short time later, having discussed the proposition in greater depth.

We felt that this would provide an opportunity to see how well Christopher would cope too, and as the other boy also had difficulty in coping in a group setting, which had been the reason behind the suggestion in the first place, sharing space on an occasional basis, might prove to be beneficial for both of them.

The plan had been implemented and following a change in circumstances, the placement had now become a permanent one. It was amusing to note that although they sometimes stood side-by-side at the sand or water trays and played with the contents quite happily, they rarely shared their pleasure of toys or activities with each other, even though they both did so with the assistants and class teacher.

Nevertheless, schooling continued to be a success as their co-existence was generally tolerated by the other child and even when one of them became agitated and irate, instead of this leading to the deterioration in their class peer, it often resulted in amused giggles and even, curiosity.

With unexpected, but continued seizure-control, respite had been successfully reintroduced earlier in the year, but had ceased a few months later. The problem this time resulted because we had been given dates, instead of regular days and when the last scheduled session had taken place no further ones had been arranged by the Social Services Department.

We had been offered 1-hour of respite every second to third week and had been asked to provide transportation to the located venue. The classroom which had been adapted for Christopher was opened by the caretaker on Wednesday evenings and as the room contained items to keep him amused, and was familiar to him, sessions had been going well. A sand and water tray had been provided by staff and the teacher had been kind enough to bring a huge paddling pool into the room which had been converted into a ball-pit. With the variety of vehicles and toys we had brought from home, there had been plenty of activities to prevent boredom and keep Christopher occupied.

It seemed ironic that with the maximum amount of effort involved in locating support workers and a suitable venue, the minimal amount of effort required to organise additional sessions had not been taken, and had resulted in it ceasing just 5 months after it had started. It had been extremely disappointing and frustrating as I had contacted the Department to request that further dates be provided weeks before the last scheduled date, but with no response to my letters, sessions had once again simply ceased.

A local solicitor had been contacted to assist us in securing respite provision, but her letters to the Director of Social Services, requesting that our complaint be addressed and appropriate provision be provided for Christopher, had been ignored. This had led her decision to contact The Local Government Ombudsman with complaints relating to the inconsistent level of respite provision and also to its inappropriate withdrawal. Following the Ombudsman's agreeing to look into the complaint, the

Council requested to complete its own independent inquiry and so, the Ombudsman withdrew having permitted them to do so.

We had been interviewed at the solicitor's office some months previously where we explained that when Christopher was displaying very high levels of aggression we were happy to cancel sessions ourselves, but we did expect support workers to manage behaviours, that the female teacher and assistants coped with for 4 hours a day. I stressed that we would be satisfied to receive 2-4 hours of respite per week, although we wished to receive additional support during holidays and that it was vital that workers had the authority to perform pad-changes during sessions, in the event that it was needed. The alternative being that we were either contacted early to collect Christopher, or he was left in a soiled/wet pad until the end of the session.

We provided documentation which detailed that respite provision had been inconsistent and often, non-existent, since it was first introduced some 5 years earlier and also provided details regarding the reasons it had ceased on each of the four occasions that it had. The interview ended a short while later and we were now awaiting the results of the investigation, without which, we could not proceed with legal action against the Council.

The bungalow was now almost complete with just the finishing touches being needed, before we were to be given the keys to move in. If the building looked enormous on paper, then in reality it was even more so and I will never forget the first moment that I walked through the front door to be shown around. The bungalow and its grounds reflected Christopher's need for safe space.

The building contained a lounge, kitchen, dining room, utility room, 3-bedrooms and a bathroom. Christopher also had an en-suite attached to his bedroom, with shower facilities and sufficient cupboard space in which to store the supply of incontinent pads which were delivered every two months.

The architect had also designed windows in the walls of several of the rooms, which would enable us to observe him whilst he wandered around his new home, without him being aware that we were doing so. In this way, he was being given *some* degree of freedom, but we could still ensure that he was safe. Furthermore, the glass in the doors and windows were either strengthened, or bullet-proof to prevent injuries from breakages.

Under-floor heating also meant that Christopher could no longer pull radiators away from the walls and sunken lights in the ceilings would prevent him from breaking bulbs when throwing objects. All of the doorways and halls were wide so that we could use his buggy indoors during the times when he refused to walk or following seizures and a stable-door had been fixed to the kitchen.

We had also requested that a stable-door be fixed to his bedroom so that we could establish a night-time routine. This would mean that when he eventually became tired, we could take him to bed and lock the lower half of the door. I didn't like the idea of closing the room completely off as we would be unable to check on him without first opening the door, so by installing our old favourite, it would prevent us from disturbing Christopher and not make him feel isolated and alone.

The bungalow was absolutely amazing and with the Welsh Assembly having passed the entire design, it also meant that a dual purpose, sensory-cum-quiet room, had been included. This room would be a place for him to retreat to when things became too much for him and also, where he could be placed for his own safety, when at his most aggressive.

This room was situated in the centre of the bungalow and its windows were positioned in such a way that they faced into the dining room, hallway and lounge. It was incredibly well thought out and when the floor and walls were covered with safety padding, it would be completed and ready to use. The padding came as sheets of foam in varying sizes, which were covered in wipe-clean durable vinyl and these would enable Christopher to simply relax, or thrash around without harming himself.

The room would also eventually contain a bubble-tube and bean-bag bed and with my sister, brother-in-law and nephews having run the London and Irish Marathons for Christopher, additional funding had also been raised to purchase a variety of equipment, including optic lights, a mirror ball, outsized foam building blocks and a large sand-pit. People's kindness in times of need never ceases to amaze me and as I looked around I realised that for the first time in Christopher's short life, he would actually have a *quality* of life and one that would not have been possible without the understanding, generosity and compassion of others.

It was a very emotional time for all of the family wondering how Christopher was going to cope in just a few weeks time, when he finally left the only home he had ever known. He did not understand that we were moving and would not initially understand that the bungalow was, in fact, his new home and we prayed that he would cope with this massive change in his young life.

Other changes had been happening too, with Michael having recently moved into his own flat. This was in the same village and although he visited most days, he would obviously not now be moving into the bungalow with us. The surveyor had assured us that this would not affect the project as it had already been passed, but it was strange to think of Michael, who was now twenty years of age, being an adult and living in his own home.

I had kept myself busy over the past few months and had painted the entire house in preparation for the move. It had always been badly affected by damp and wall-paper rarely stayed up, but we wanted to leave it looking as good as it could for the next residents. And so, with sixteen years of memories finally packed, there was nothing left for us to do, but wait until the moving date.

Having asked if it was possible for us to name the bungalow and been given permission to do so, we had wanted to give it a fitting title for this momentous occasion in all of our lives. I recalled how the same phrase came into my mind whenever I considered the move, as it filled us with renewed hope for the future.

On 17th September 2004 and armed with boxes of varying sizes, we glanced across at the wood and ceramic house plaque which had been secured to the fence and smiled – Dechrau Newydd – new start/new beginning. We were exhausted, but ecstatic and realised that for the first time in nine years we would once again be sleeping in a proper bed. It seemed such a silly thing to remark upon and yet, as we closed the front door behind us, we could think of nothing more that we would prefer to do.

……………

CHAPTER FOURTEEN

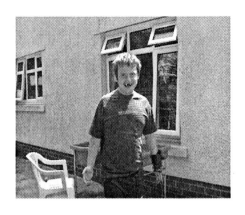

Christopher aged 16 years

We had lived in our new home for a few months now, but it was still strange to imagine that this would be the last one that we would ever share together as a family. Having been at school that day in September, Christopher had simply walked through the front door then jumped straight onto the sofa exhausted. We had waited for the confusion and distress to set in but there had been nothing but acceptance. He could be a real puzzle at times, but our relief at his reaction was unimaginable. He had been a real star.

We had established a bed-time routine with no objection and from the first night he had climbed into bed as if it was an action he was well accustomed to making. He was not able to pull the bedding over him with any real accuracy, but by folding the duvet into three pleats so that it rested against the foot-rest, we realised that he was able to pull the edge upwards, which resulted in him mostly being covered. If he moved and the duvet slipped, he could not straighten it and pull it over himself again, but having managed to complete the first part of the manoeuvre, it seemed probable that over time he would also work out how to do the latter.

If Christopher was displaying any obvious signs of tiredness we would lead him to his bedroom, help him into bed then wait to see if he would settle. If he was happy to remain in the room but had climbed out of bed, then we encouraged him to remain where he was, by distracting him with balls and cars from his toy-box. If this didn't work, then we resorted to placing cartoons on his television-DVD and would either turn the volume low or off altogether. Mostly one of these distraction-techniques worked, but if Christopher would not settle and became distressed then we re-opened the stable-door, allowed him to wander around and repeated the whole process again when he became noticeably tired.

Having placed heavy duty fasteners on some of the doors, such as bathroom, utility, kitchen, en-suite, etc, to prevent him from gaining access, he was able to wander around without many difficulties arising. We had spent so many years shadowing him that it seemed unnatural to sit down and relax and it had taken several weeks of realising that he could not come to any harm before we allowed him to roam around on his own. Of course, this was the reason the bungalow had been built and the reason the criteria had been so strict, but our confidence in his surroundings had to be absolute and this had taken time.

The meal-time routine had also gone exceptionally well and Christopher would sometimes sit at the table throughout an entire meal. The staff at school had worked tremendously hard to establish this skill and he could now take a loaded spoon to his mouth when he was calm enough to do so. If the meal was sloppy, then more assistance was needed, but when the food was tacky and stuck to the spoon then there were very little spillages. Christopher could also take a loaded fork to his mouth, and he was becoming more tolerant with our attempts to assist him in loading the cutlery.

There were days when he was too aggressive to assist with feeding and so we would feed him over the stable-door and of course, there were still occasions when he would attempt to throw food and crockery – even when he was in a mischievous-type of mood, but substantial progress had still been made and for this, we were grateful.

With the continued use of stinted sentences he also now recognised the term *pad-change* and when he was amiable he would come to the bedroom when called so that we could complete this task. We supported his weight while we lay him down on the floor to clean him, as this was still the only position which we had found that enabled us to do a thorough enough job, and infrequently he would lie down by himself, asking in his own way for the pad to be removed.

However, probably the most significant improvement regarded the use of objects. We had bought plastic plates and beakers prior to the move, with the intention of using Velcro to stick them on to the wall. We hoped that if the items were in sight then Christopher might learn to collect a plate or beaker and bring it to us if we were out of the room. He would already do so if we were nearby, but we hoped he would progress to carrying the item to wherever we happened to be.

But without even being shown what was expected of him, Christopher began to collect the plate or beaker and would wander from room to room until he found either Philip or me. He would then offer the object and follow us to the kitchen where he would wait until the requested drink or meal was made for him.

Although we continued to use objects and progress was being made, we were disappointed to learn that staff at school had introduced PECS some months earlier without our knowledge. During our first meeting with the teacher we had advised that the system had previously been used and discarded in favour of objects of reference. And this information was also contained in the past Statements I had provided along with the psychiatrist's advice, but unfortunately it had not been heeded.

Having previously reached the stage where he would offer a card unprompted, Christopher quickly remembered the procedure and it was difficult to make it understood that he was *not* learning the system from new, but had already been taught it years earlier. The staff appeared to have forgotten that he was acquainted with the use of the cards and were encouraged by his rapid understanding of what to do. But although we again stressed that as he still did not take any interest in pictures it seemed unlikely that he would progress any further than he had previously, their efforts continued.

Although we doubted that progress would be made we supported the staff nonetheless and accepted the offered cards to use at home. The pictures were line-drawings and not photographs of actual brands and we realised that they would have no meaning for Christopher. We wondered if we might have more success laminating packets which were familiar to him, as although they would be much larger to begin with they could eventually be downsized over time and we decided to give it a try.

It was amazing how he could recognise a flattish empty packet, but could not recognise that same packet in a laminated sheet. It looked almost identical to Philip and me, but although he would use the card, he never glanced down at it and as the months turned into a year, with no improvements forthcoming we asked that objects once again be used instead. We felt that PECS had been given a fair enough trial on both of the occasions it had been used and that progress with Christopher's ability to communicate should be given priority over any personal preference which the staff or ourselves might have.

It was recognised and accepted that he was still not able to differentiate between the pictures on the cards and an agreement was made to introduce objects of reference instead, but staff asked if the cards could be used alongside of objects and this compromise was reached. We supplied the school with a small lunch-box, plastic beaker, plastic plate, etc, so that Christopher could use the preferred item to convey his wishes in the classroom. Once the item was presented to staff, the equivalent could be collected from his bag and offered.

The dual method appeared to work for a while and PECS was primarily used to request individual crisps at break time each day. This provided Christopher with the opportunity to interact with the person completing the session and also provided him with an activity which would keep him occupied for a set amount of time. This was particularly useful during the occasions when he was in one of his eating phases and he initially accepted the use of both systems without objection.

However, we were concerned to learn that he was once again resorting to offering unrelated items and becoming agitated when we failed to guess correctly what was being requested. More worrying still was that familiar objects which had only ever had one meaning for Christopher were also being used as a *ticket* as well as for requesting the related food or activity.

If we happened to fill his cup when he had offered it but he had not been requesting a drink, then he would throw it at us or at the walls. The difficulty being that there were occasions when he offered the cup *wanting* it refilled, but we never knew when this was the case or if he was simply asking for something different.

He began to pass shoes or keys and then became aggressive if we led him to the front door and more aggressive whilst we offered unwanted items when we realised that our initial guess had been wrong. He had struggled to find a way to communicate all those years ago and had done so well, but suddenly we were unable to understand what was wanted and it was distressing for all involved.

Having supplied all the information I had, only to be ignored, left me feeling upset and angry on his behalf. Not only had the re-introduction and continued use of PECS prevented Christopher from progressing using objects of reference, but it had set him back years. We no longer knew what he was requesting and he no longer knew how to make his wishes known.

We immediately asked that PECS be withdrawn altogether having explained the difficulties its use had caused and although this was done without delay, we worried about how long it would take for him to regain his skills of using objects appropriately, or if he ever would.

The deterioration in Christopher's ability to communicate was disappointing, but with Social Services having located a centre where future respite sessions could take place the situation was made more bearable. The social worker and occupational therapist arrived to complete a risk assessment regarding the issue of transportation as having provided our vehicle to past workers or driven Christopher ourselves, we had written to the Department stating that we now wished for them to take responsibility for the task.

We did not wish to be left without a vehicle again whilst the support workers used it and if we had agreed to drive Christopher to the centre then it would impact upon the few conditional hours we were to receive or affect what we were able to do. We had always compromised in the past, believing that any restrictions would only be temporary, but things had never improved. The purpose of respite was to provide carers with the chance to relax and recharge their batteries, not place additional demands and conditions on them. And yet, as I sat listening to the occupational therapist's proposals, I wondered why I had written to the Department, as the conditions and restrictions appeared to be even worse than they had previously been.

Firstly, we had to demonstrate to the workers how to use the travel harness and as it was accepted that Christopher would then believe that he was going out for a drive, we would have to do so. Philip would drive, I was to sit in the front passenger seat and one of the support workers would sit alongside of Christopher in the back passenger seat. We were expected to repeat this first stage each session until the support worker felt confident enough to do it alone.

When this stage had been achieved the roles would be reversed, so instead of one of the support workers sitting alongside of Christopher in the back of the vehicle, Philip or I would have to do so, which meant that the driving would then be done by the support worker instead. Again, this whole procedure would be completed each session until the support worker felt confident enough to do it without assistance. At a later point it was hoped that a taxi with wheelchair access could be used, but as Christopher had a buggy and not a standard wheelchair, the social worker was unsure whether the clamps in the taxi would fit onto the smaller wheels.

The third stage involved us driving to the actual venue and once again Philip or I would have to accompany him each week, until the support workers were confident to progress to the next stage. This involved taking him out from the vehicle at the centre, placing him in his buggy and pushing him into the room which he would be using. One parent would also be needed for this.

In addition to the other stages, the fifth stage involved him completing a session with the two support workers, but Philip or I would need to be present until the six and final stage had been reached, which meant that the support workers would complete everything themselves and we would not be required to do anything – except, collect him if he deteriorated whilst there. Although the occupational therapist stated that even after completing the procedure, the risks involved might be considered to be too high and would therefore not come in to fruition.

I wondered how long all of this was going to go on for before we actually received the respite we had been promised. We would still be expected to cancel sessions which meant that each stage would take longer to reach and Christopher's behaviour was always unpredictable. He might be excellent for two sessions and aggressive for the next and then where would that leave us?

The social worker then mentioned that it was hoped we could be offered two sessions each week, but one of those would be scheduled for Saturdays when the centre was not open. Suddenly I knew what was coming. We had been asked on several occasions if the workers could use the spare bedroom as a venue as there was some confusion on the Department's part as to its original purpose.

Having been advised that it had been designed for respite purposes by the Leader of Children with

Disabilities Team, we had contacted the architect and surveyor to ask that they clarify the situation with the Department and they had since done so. The room had been intended for Michael who had been living at home when the architect had designed it, but following the Assembly's approval, he had moved into his own flat. The room was only 10 feet x 10 feet in any event and having allowed Christopher to roam freely around since we had first moved in would only cause difficulties and confusion if he was restricted in such a small space. Nevertheless the anticipated request came and I was again asked to speak with Philip.

But having discussed it at length our minds remained unchanged. I would have had to remain at home until the workers were confident to be left in charge of Christopher and then we would have to leave the bungalow for sessions to take place. It was nice to be able to go out if we *chose* to, but being told we *had* to, when we might have otherwise chosen to catch up on sleep or complete chores around the home, was no respite. We contacted the Department to advise of our decision stating that we did not wish to have sessions provided at home, but we agreed to visit the proposed centre so that we could view the room.

It was an amazing building and because it was used by disabled adults the rooms were huge and the corridors were wide to cater for wheelchair access. The centre's bathroom was equipped with pad-changing facilities and there was also a beautiful sensory room which we were told Christopher could use. The proposed room was also impressive and provided ample space so that he could run around without hurting himself. I was delighted and immediately accepted the offer.

Unfortunately, it was at this point that the manager explained that the centre would be transferring over to the Education Department by the end of the year. The remark came as a huge blow to the social worker and occupational therapist who had evidently not been informed of this fact. It also now meant that our wait to receive practical support was once again delayed as the search for another venue continued.

CHAPTER FIFTEEN

....

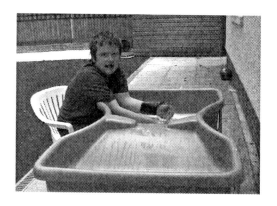

Christopher aged 17 years

Since the proposed centre had fallen through some months previously, the Social Services Department had not had any success in locating another venue. This meant that we were still without practical support although the Department had made some progress by locating a second male support worker to provide support for Christopher.

Support workers had always come in pairs although Christopher had typically been allocated two female workers in the past. It was therefore reassuring to learn that when the service was eventually reintroduced at some later date, the additional strength which the male workers would provide would prevent them from feeling so intimidated by Christopher's own size and strength.

Things appeared to be headed in the right direction, but we had been without any respite services for over a year and although the Independent Investigator had now completed his report, we had been further disappointed to learn that our complaints against the Council had not been upheld. We were surprised by the reasons given, as we felt that we had proven our complaints against the Council had been justified and as we read through the findings we were also somewhat confused by the decision.

The first complaint of '*inconsistent respite provision*' had been rejected, because, in the Investigator's opinion, Social Services had made great efforts in trying to provide services to Christopher. The fact that their efforts did not *actually* result in us receiving any respite, was not in dispute, but it seemed to make little difference to his opinion. The number of occasions respite had ceased was not even included in the report, nor the duration of time we had been left without respite whenever it had ceased and as these details would have proven that respite had been inconsistent, it seemed totally illogical that they had been omitted.

The second complaint was that '*the withdrawal of the service whenever it had been withdrawn had not been appropriate*' but this had also been rejected because the Investigator stated that it had been a health and safety issue. However, respite had ceased on 4 separate occasions, but behavioural difficulties had only been an issue on 1 of those occasions. There was *no* mention that we had been left without a service when Social Services had failed to replace support workers who were leaving, *or* that they had failed to provide additional dates to sessions that were going well which again resulted in us being left without a service. These omissions tended to lead the reader to believe that respite had *always* ceased because of behavioural difficulties, which simply wasn't true.

As I continued to read through the report I noticed that it contained several discrepancies, particularly with regards to the amount of respite to which we had been provided. Also, as there was no mention of services ceasing on some of the occasions, it gave the impression that respite had been on-going, at times when we had not actually been receiving any practical support.

I wondered where the Independent Investigator had got some of the information from and why he had not studied Christopher's file to ensure that the details were correct before committing himself. I was suddenly relieved that I had always kept past correspondence between ourselves and the Department so that we would be able to prove the inaccuracies. …And, having glanced at the letter which had accompanied the report, I decided to contact the Assistant Director of Social Services to do so.

I also contacted the solicitor for advice as we were not satisfied with the report or its findings and a short time later we were informed that a Stage 3 Complaint was the final stage of the Council's own complaints procedure and that arrangements had therefore been made for us to proceed to this level. Unfortunately, we were also advised that legal aid could not be applied for to fund the solicitor's presence at the hearing and, as we did not have sufficient funds to pay for her presence ourselves, we were advised to make notes during the meeting which could be sent to her office afterwards.

Home-life was stressful and fighting to secure yet another service left its toll. We seemed forever to be battling one cause or another and instead of Social Services providing a care-package which reflected Christopher's complex needs, they had repeatedly used it as a reason not to do so. It was exhausting and with the deterioration of Christopher's behaviour once again, we found ourselves alone and under even more pressure.

The aggression which had been infrequent up until recently slowly began to worsen and school was once again cancelled on a regular basis. Christopher rarely completed a full week and most weeks he attended school for just one or two days. We continued to carry our mobile phone around although we were seldom contacted by staff to collect him as we simply kept him home if he was displaying any aggression in the mornings.

We were not overly concerned at first as Christopher always presented with several days of medium-higher levels of aggression every month, but when several weeks had passed with no improvement, we began to wonder if he was in any way ill. The psychiatrist made a visit and advised that the severity of his aggression might suggest that he was in pain and having noticed that Christopher had begun to bite and clamp his teeth down on surfaces and clothing, we dreaded that there might be a problem with his teeth

The community nurse was contacted and arrangements were made for a dentist to call on us at home to examine Christopher and having harnessed him in his buggy, Philip, Michael and I restrained his arms and head so that the dentist could look inside his mouth. The dentist was un-phased by the situation and despite warnings that he would bite down to the bone if given the opportunity; she completed the examination cautiously but professionally.

The news was not what we wanted to hear. Christopher had abscesses over the teeth either side of his existing gap which would need removing under general anaesthetic. The memories came flooding back from our last hospital visit and all I could think of is how on earth we were going to restrain him and keep him safe in a hospital room at his current size. The dentist assured us that staff were well accustomed to carrying out surgery on patients with challenging behaviour, but how often had we been assured the same thing only to later discover that there was a limit to the challenges which professionals could deal with.

Christopher was given a prescription and the dentist advised that she would make the necessary arrangements at the local hospital. Oral surgery was scheduled for every second Wednesday and it was hoped that the teeth extraction could be completed within just a few days. However, a fault with the equipment meant that he had to wait a further two weeks and a stronger antibiotic was prescribed to be administered after the first course had been completed.

A few days before he was due to attend hospital we were contacted by the dentist to advise us of the procedure which was to be followed. Staff would prepare a separate waiting room near to the theatre, but away from other patients and as sedation had previously proved to be unsuccessful, it would not be given. Christopher could be wheeled into the theatre in his buggy and the anaesthetist would remove the mask from the pipe and hold this under his nose instead.

He could then be lifted out from his buggy and placed onto the trolley by Philip and Michael. He would be given the minimal amount of time required to recover following the extractions and he would be allowed to return home as soon as possible. Although in theory this procedure not only sounded *acceptable*, but *exceptional*, past experience still meant that we were doubtful as to whether this would actually happen on the day itself.

We arrived at the hospital on the scheduled date feeling more than a little apprehensive as we parked the car and harnessed Christopher into his buggy. We were relieved that he would finally be receiving treatment he needed, but also feeling somewhat guilty as Christopher evidently assumed that he was going on an outing. Surprisingly, he was in a lovely mood and with the letter clutched in my hand, we made our way to the area where oral surgery was performed.

As we scanned the information placards for further details, a lady suddenly took an interest in us and we realised that we had been fortunate enough to meet a nurse from the same Department who was arriving to begin her own shift. She led us through the maze of corridors and then into the agreed separate waiting room where we were left to settle in. Shortly after our arrival another nurse entered and having introduced herself asked if the necessary medical questionnaire could be completed away from Christopher, to prevent any distress. Michael offered to remain in the room with his brother so that Philip could accompany me and we were shown into a smaller room a short distance away.

The relevant details were taken down and just as the questionnaire was nearing completion the consultant dentist entered with a parental consent form which needed to be filled in. This new form was required because Christopher was over 16 years of age but could not make decisions for himself.

The dentist advised that there would be no attempts made to perform any pre-op observations to avoid any distress. She also advised that she would be happy to remove any additional teeth because of the circumstances we were in and although we were initially tempted, we felt that he had gone through enough the past few months and so we decided against the offer.

When the form had been dated and signed, we returned to the waiting room to await the arrival of the doctor. Soon afterwards Philip and Michael wheeled Christopher down to theatre as agreed and whilst they were absent a nurse showed me to the recovery room where she mentioned that he would remain after surgery for up to 10 minutes. I was then taken back to the waiting room where I was joined by Philip and Michael. Philip mentioned that additional theatre staff had waited outside of the theatre until Christopher had been placed under anaesthetic to avoid upset.

Everything was running as smoothly as the dentist had stated that it would, but we were still waiting for problems to arise. Around 20 minutes had elapsed when a nurse came hurrying into the waiting room to collect the buggy, which Philip had wheeled back after placing him on the trolley. We were advised that he was coming around and asked to accompany her to assist.

As we entered the recovery room it was to see Christopher looking exhausted, but already attempting to sit up on the trolley. The anaesthetist was tapping his shoulder reassuringly and talking to him and when Christopher attempted to climb down, the dentist decided to remove the drip which had been attached to his hand to avoid injury.

Christopher was once again restrained in his buggy, but as he was now fully awake we were advised that he could return to the waiting room for a short time. I was taken outside to receive the necessary guidelines regarding potential difficulties and before the nurse had completed this brief discussion, he had been discharged.

We were absolutely stunned. *Everything* had been prepared, *everyone* had been informed of the procedure and the staff had shown compassion and an understanding befitting of their roles. They had been brilliant and on returning home, Christopher immediately ran to the kitchen to request an angel delight. That evening we received the first kisses and cuddles we had for several weeks.

....

CHAPTER SIXTEEN

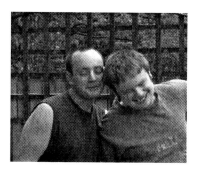

Michael with Christopher aged 17 years

Following the operation to remove his teeth Christopher had once again settled and with the re-introduction of respite in September 2005 things were once again beginning to improve. We had been offered 2-hourly sessions and provided with 3 months of dates with a promise of further ones. The sessions were currently being held in our local community hall and as the venue was within minutes of our home, we had agreed to provide transportation.

We had been a little disappointed to have had dates provided once again instead of regular days, as this meant that sessions were irregular. Some weeks we received a maximum of 2 sessions, some weeks 1 session and some weeks we received no respite at all, but at least we were receiving some practical support even if it was, once again, on a conditional basis.

The support workers were not able to complete pad-changes during the sessions, but as we hoped that this would be addressed during the Stage 3 Complaint, we accepted that in the meantime there would be occasions when we would be contacted early. We also accepted that as the hall had no play-facilities we would have to take toys each session, but again, we were hoping that this issue would be addressed during the complaints procedure.

A date for the hearing had already been scheduled and cancelled some months previously as one of the Council's representatives would not have been able to attend, but a new date had now been arranged. We had originally assumed that the purpose of the hearing was to have our original complaints re-examined, as a type of second opinion, and had therefore been somewhat confused to learn that the Stage 2 report would be under scrutiny, along with its contents and decisions and not the complaints themselves.

With no knowledge of what the procedure would entail, or how we were meant to prepare our summary, I had sat at the computer for hours at a time examining the report and trying to work out what information I should include. Philip had contacted several agencies in the hope that they could provide some assistance, but as soon as he mentioned that a solicitor was involved, none would offer support even though he stated that the solicitor would not be present at the actual hearing. Nevertheless, Philip had ploughed on with pen and pad in hand, striking off any negative responses and moving on to other possibilities.

Eventually his efforts had paid off when he had located an advocacy worker, who had not only agreed to help us prepare for the hearing, but who would also attend. The only drawback being, that he felt it best that I continued to represent our case, as he would not be able to answer any questions which might be put to him by the Panel. It was a bit of a disappointment, but at least with his knowledge of how the procedure worked, I would not embarrass myself.

We had learned that there would be 8 people present at the hearing - 3 members of the Panel, the clerk, 2 Social Services employees, the senior council solicitor and the Independent Investigator who had been responsible for completing the Stage 2 report. And of course, there would also now be the advocacy worker, Philip and me.

The thought of standing before so many people had made me feel physically sick for the past few weeks and since having learned that the Council would be represented by its own solicitor, made the prospect of outlining our case against them seem even more intimidating than it already was. It seemed unfair and placed us at a distinct disadvantage, but we were grateful that the advocacy worker had experience of such hearings and was able to offer such sound advice.

Although I had contacted the Assistant Director of Social Services some months previously to request that the Stage 2 report be amended, no corrections had been made and having learned that the Panel was going to be sent copies of the report, I had contacted the Independent Investigator with the same request. I had been extremely concerned that a decision might, in part be made, on the inaccurate information which had been supplied but although the Investigator had responded to my letter, it was simply to state that my comments had been noted.

Having then sought advice from the advocacy worker who was shown the documents and correspondence, I had been advised to send copies of this additional information to the council solicitor and request that it be sent to the Panel Members so that it could be included in the bundle.

In addition to these documents I had also sent copies of information that we had been sent by CEREBRA – The Foundation for the Brain Injured Infant, which detailed our legal entitlements to receive services for Christopher *irrespective* of the level of challenge he presented with. I didn't feel that there would be any difficulty in proving that respite had been inappropriately withdrawn on 3 occasions, but as the fourth related to health and safety, I wasn't sure if the Panel would be aware that Social Services had a legal obligation to provide practical support.

I thought back to the psychologist's report which had been completed a few years earlier and decided that I would also include this as the opinion completely differed to that of the independent investigator. The sentence *'exceptional difficulties, should have resulted in an exceptional response and not a response that effectively says, Christopher's case is too complex for Social Services to support'*, still stayed firmly in my mind.

As I glanced down at the guidelines that we had been sent regarding the procedure for the hearing, I felt the panic once again set in:

1   The Chairman introduces the Panel, The Clerk, The Council's Representative and the Complainant.

2   The Chairman explains the procedure.

3   The Complainant's representative outlines their case and calls any witnesses.
4   The Council's representative asks questions to the Complainant's Representative and any witnesses.
5   The Members of the Panel ask questions to the Complainant's Representative's and any witnesses.
6   The Council outlines their case and calls any witnesses.
7   The Complainant's representative asks questions to the Council's representative and any witnesses.
8   The Members of the Panel ask questions to the Council's representative and any witnesses.
9   The Complainant's representative sums up.
10   The Council's representative sums up.
11   The Complainant's representative and the Council's representative leave the room.
12   The Panel consider its decision taking advice from the Clerk.
13   A written copy of the decision to be sent in writing to the Complainant's representative and to the Council's representative.

My hands shook as I leafed through the notes that I had made and would be reading through. The advocacy worker had suggested that by making copies for each person at the hearing, it would ensure that people would not be looking directly at me, but would instead be reading along with me. This particular piece of advice had been gratefully received and would also mean that the Panel Members would not need to make notes whilst I outlined our case, which should speed up the hearing.

I had read through the notes several times each day, hoping that I would make less errors if I familiarised myself with them, but as I sat upon the edge of the bed I found myself repeating the process once again......

.....*'Following the Stage 2 investigation conducted by (name) we requested a review panel hearing as we were not satisfied with either the content of the report or its findings.*

'We do not believe that the decisions reached by the report were reached fairly. We also believe that there are several contradictions between the report and the letters we received from Social Services both prior to, and following (name) investigation.

1)   *Unfairness*

*The decisions reached in the stage 2 report were arrived at without properly assessing our claim that **the Council has failed to provide a consistent level of respite care** for Christopher.*

From 1998 – 2004 we accessed respite services and during that time respite has ceased on 4 separate occasions. On each of the occasions when respite ceased, our family were left without services from durations ranging from several months to over a year.

Details regarding the duration of time our family has been left without respite services whenever it has ceased, were not included in the report although details of which are prevalent to our first complaint.

*The decisions reached in the stage 2 report were arrived at without properly assessing our claim that **the reason for the withdrawal of the service whenever it has been withdrawn, are not appropriate.***

On the 1st occasion respite ceased when new support workers were not located to replace the ones who were leaving – we do not believe that this is an appropriate reason for respite services to have ceased.

On the 3rd occasion respite ceased due to an increase in the seizures Christopher was experiencing – we do believe that this was an appropriate reason for respite to have ceased and was unavoidable given the circumstances.

On the 4th occasion respite ceased when no additional dates for sessions were organised during the Social Worker's absence on maternity leave – we do not believe that this was an appropriate reason for respite to have ceased.

And yet, the only reason concentrated on in the report was when the respite services were withdrawn for health and safety reasons on the 2nd occasion. With regards to this particular issue, we refer you to the decision of the High Court in B v East Sussex County Council (2003) where it was held that a service should not be withdrawn under a 'no risk' elimination' regime, but rather a 'risk reduction' or 'risk minimisation' programme should be in use in order that the individual may be able to continue to receive services.

We believe that (borough name) Social Services did in fact withdraw their service without satisfactorily exploring any 'risk reduction' or 'risk minimisation' strategy. Services should not have been withdrawn for Health and Safety reasons. Social Services should have had access to suitably trained individuals who could manage Christopher's challenging behaviour.

We refer to the legal guidance we passed to Social Services from Cerebra, The Foundation for the Brain Injured Infant.

Under the heading, 'Community Care/Law and Guidance', it states that 'the fact that Christopher has challenging behaviour does not legally justify the reduction or rationing of services…in fact the opposite is true, challenging behaviour usually requires additional services. To make respite care conditional to 'good behaviour' on the grounds of health and safety, is therefore turning the law on its head.'

The legal guidance we have received clearly states that those who present with challenging behaviour should in fact be offered greater support rather than services being suspended. We therefore do not believe that withdrawing respite for health and safety reasons was an appropriate reason for respite to cease.

2   **<u>Unfairness and Human Rights</u>**

Our opinion is that (borough's name) failure to provide adequate respite care infringes Christopher's Human Rights and is thus unlawful.

This part of our complaint was not addressed in Mr (name) report. We consider the stage 2 investigation flawed because it did not consider this issue.

We consider (borough's) Social Services to be in breach of The Children's Act 1989, (Schedule 2, part 1); this states that in paragraph 6,

'Every local authority should give (disabled children) the opportunity to lead lives which are as normal as possible'.

We believe that the Council has broken its promise in this duty in its failure to provide adequate respite care and the random withdrawal of respite care.

Furthermore paragraph 8 of the act states that,

'Every local authority shall make such provision as they consider appropriate for the following services to be available with respect to children in need while they are living with their families.

d) facilities for, or assistance with, travelling to and from home for the purpose of taking advantage of any other service provided under this act or any similar service.'

We do not believe that Social Services have complied with this requirement. We believe that Christopher has been discriminated against pursuant to the Disability Discrimination Act 1995 in relation to the transport to and from respite care.

This is further backed up by the Disabled Person's Act 1970 Section 2(1). This states that a local authority has a duty to provide transport to and from educational facilities, day services and community activities.

We consider that Christopher's Human Rights have been breached as the UN Convention on Human Rights has not been observed. Article 23 recognises the disabled child's right to,

'Enjoy a full and decent life, in conditions that ensure dignity, promote self reliance, and facilitate the child's active participation in the community.'

By failing to provide adequate and consistent levels of respite, and by Social Services attempting to justify respite in the home rather than in the community, we believe that (borough name) to be in breach of Article 23.

We consider that Christopher should be given the opportunity to integrate with others away from his home environment and enjoy activities that may be other than those he is engaged in during school.....'

Part 3 of my notes detailed the errors which had been contained in the report and finally, my comments regarding the Investigator's mention of budgetary implications when providing services to Christopher. It appeared to have covered all eventualities and I hoped that all of our hard work during the past few weeks would at least mean that we put up a worthy fight.

....

Having dropped Christopher off at school to begin his schooling at 10.00am we drove the few miles to the proposed venue. I scanned the cars outside to see if the advocacy worker's was among them, but there were too many and with the hearing due to start in the next ten minutes we rushed up the steps and hoped that he was already there.

I was relieved to notice that he was already waiting in the reception area for our arrival and as we entered the building, he led the way upstairs to the room which was being used for the hearing. Representatives from the Social Services Department were already seated in the waiting area and we were informed that the Panel was preparing the room for our arrival.

It all suddenly seemed very unreal as we sat there waiting to be summoned by the Clerk and although Philip and I were very nervous about the prospect of the hearing - where we would be seated in the same room as the very people we were complaining about – the Social Services employees seemed relaxed and amiable.

A few moments later the spokesman of the Panel joined us and asked if there was any objection to Philip and me meeting with the rest of the Panel first, and this being agreed we followed him into the room and made the necessary introductions. A few moments later, the rest of the party joined us and I was then asked to outline our case.

I passed around the copies I had prepared for the meeting and was relieved to note that not only were they accepted, but were appreciated by the Panel. I was immensely nervous despite the endless repetitions and made a few minor stumbles throughout the summary, but although my voice trembled on occasions, as I finished my speech, I felt pleased with my effort.

A brief pause ensued before the spokesperson addressed the Independent Investigator and asked if he would reconsider his decision regarding the issue of inconsistent provision. I was dismayed to hear the decisive 'no' given in response to the question, having provided details in the summary of the occasions we had been left without any services and also, details regarding the duration of the gaps in provision between respite ceasing and then recommencing. He continued that the Department had made great efforts in their attempts to provide practical support and had detailed accounts of these efforts on file and so, in his opinion, the Department could have done nothing further.

The spokesperson reiterated the gaps in provision I had mentioned and asked again if, in his opinion, respite services had been inconsistent, but was met with a response relating to the Council not having a legal duty to provide a service to Christopher. He again stated that the Department had made great efforts in attempting to reinstate services.

The spokesperson stated that the efforts the Department had placed into securing services was not the basis of the complaint, but rather that its efforts had not resulted in a consistent level of respite service and when pressed once more, the Investigator stated that in that case he would uphold our first complaint. The atmosphere in the room was electric, but although this sudden change of opinion was a much welcome surprise, the feeling of unease remained as I wondered what questions might yet be put to us.

Now that the first complaint had been dealt with, a second Panel Member addressed the Investigator and asked if he had read the copy of the decision of the High Court in B v East Sussex County Council 2003 which had been sent to every Council following the ruling. As this was the information that CEREBRA had originally sent to me, and which I had in turn sent to the Panel, I was very interested in the response.

The Panel Member continued that providing a service to the complainant had never been an issue of contention with the ruling. The decision had been that the Council was to minimise and reduce risks so that the complainant could receive a service and not to weigh up the risks to decide if a service could be offered, as the Investigator appeared to believe.

The spokesperson then asked the Team Leader, of Children with Disabilities Team, where the risk assessments were regarding the issue when respite had been withdrawn for health and safety reasons, as they were not contained within the bundle and following some discussion we learned that no assessments had been devised on how risks could have been minimised during transportation.

The Investigator was then asked where the details were regarding our initial complaint as the bundle contained no clear account of what action had been undertaken following our first complaint and the Stage 2 Complaint report. Despite our letters to our local Assembly Member, and her resulting letter to the Director of Social Services, the Investigator stated that this did not constitute a complaint. When I asked would a letter from our solicitor be regarded as one, I was met with a reluctant response in the affirmative.

The Panel Member then informed the Investigator that it was not only his responsibility, to clarify these points, but to ensure that the details in the bundle were correct before submitting them for consideration.

The hearing continued in much the same way and as it came to a close, the only question we had been asked by the Panel was if we were satisfied with the 4-hours of weekly respite we had been offered. Having made so much progress during the past 1½ hours I declined to mention that the hours fluctuated from week to week and simply answered that we were.

I could hardly believe that despite our fears and ignorance of such procedures, we had obviously been very well prepared, whilst the Council's representatives had been unable to answer questions put to them and did not have details in their files that they were evidently expected to have.

Following the summing up we shook hands with the Panel Members and prepared to leave for the short journey home. It was still only late morning, but I felt completely exhausted as we said our farewells to the advocacy worker who had supported us during the past few weeks.

We were optimistic that the first complaint would now be upheld, but although the implications regarding the High Court ruling in the East Sussex case were positive, the risks involved were not related to challenging behaviour and we wondered if this would affect the Panel's decision.

CHAPTER SEVENTEEN

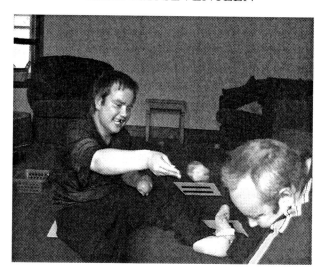

Christopher aged 18 years

It had been some weeks since the Complaint hearing and although we were feeling quietly optimistic of the outcome, we found ourselves completely unprepared when the letter actually arrived in the post. We thought back to the years it had taken before we had been offered any services after requesting them, to the months and years in between provision and to the interview we had been summoned to at the Social Services Department, following its withdrawal and we wondered if things would ever improve.

The implications of our success would be immense, as it would mean no more excuses from the

Department. They would have to offer unconditional respite, which would mean no more telephone calls during sessions requesting that we collect Christopher early, no more cancellations due to worker absence and no more excuses with regards to non-existent venues.

As Philip opened the letter I waited in silence. I watched as his eyes moved along each line, but as he never read letters aloud, I knew that it was pointless asking any questions until he had completely finished. His expression gave nothing away as he finally held the papers out for me, but as I accepted them I noticed that he was smiling...

With regards to the investigation, the Panel was of the opinion that the Stage 2 report should have contained details of the attempts made by the Council to continue to restore the respite service once it had ceased. The Panel felt that although the attempts made by the Council had been a significant factor for the Independent Investigator to have reached his conclusions, the opinion was not supported in the report by satisfactory evidence.

The Panel did not consider that the Stage 2 report addressed sufficiently all of the instances of withdrawal of the respite service as there was no mention of any reason for withdrawal, other than when services had ceased for health and safety reasons on the second occasion.   The report should have described each instance when respite had ceased and also supplied the reason it had ceased.

The Panel stated that it did not understand why the Stage 2 Investigator had reached the conclusions he had. With the evidence of withdrawals detailed in our own summary, it was felt that the only reasonable conclusion to have been reached for the first complaint was that there had not been a consistent level of provision of respite service. The Panel therefore felt that our complaint should have been upheld.

As regards to the second complaint the Panel advised that the Stage 2 report should have described the health and safety risks which had been identified as being the reason for the withdrawal of the respite service in July 2002. The report should have also specified who identified those risks.

As I read the next paragraph, I felt a growing optimism for the outcome of the second complaint. The Panel stated that the Investigator had been mistaken in his understanding of the East Sussex case, as the case indicated that the Council needed to assess the service user's needs, strike a balance between the assessments and, where necessary, take all appropriate steps to minimise the risks. Not, as the Investigator had thought, that the Council had to decide whether or not to provide a service.

The Panel stated that they had been shown no evidence that the Council had adopted the correct approach in seeking to balance risks and needs, and, in particular, they felt that the Council took no cognisance of the code issued to all local authorities by the Disability Rights Commission following the East Sussex judgment.

Since the Stage 2 report indicated that the reasons for withdrawal related to health and safety issues, the Panel considered that the Investigator's conclusion was not one which could reasonably have been reached.

It was recommended that the Council send a written apology to our family for their failure to provide a consistent level of respite care and, when such care was not being provided, for the failure to provide an adequate reason. That the Council should be clear when using the term 'resources' as it had been assumed that the meaning was a financial resource and not physical resources which had later been corrected. And finally, that the Council should give guidance to Independent Investigators which should include the need for interviewees to be sent a copy of their interview record to check for accuracy and where appropriate, for the Investigator to include his/her report recommendations to the Council....

We had done it! Our complaints had been upheld on both parts and all of the work we had placed into organising our case during the past few months had finally been worthwhile. We contacted the family to share our good news and then the advocacy worker, who had been an invaluable source of support in helping us prepare our case for the hearing. For four years we had fought to receive services and as we read the Panel's report through again, my relief came in the form of tears. It was like being on an emotional rollercoaster. One minute we were struggling to cope in sometimes, horrendous circumstances and the next; we were being offered a much needed life-line.

Our lives had taken many twists and turns since we had first discovered that Christopher was profoundly disabled, some sixteen and half years ago. Looking back, I don't believe that we truly understood the impact his disabilities would have on our lives, and we certainly did not understand how much we would learn from him, and grow from our experiences.

The love that I feel when I look into his eyes is beyond description and the pride I feel when he accomplishes even the smallest achievement is immense. He has taught us so many things in his short life, not least compassion, understanding, and awareness that not everyone is fortunate enough to have a good quality of life. We are determined to do our utmost to ensure that Christopher enjoys his.

. . . .

IN CONCLUSION

As I write this, and despite the Panel's recommendations following the Stage 3 Complaint hearing, no progress has been made. Our last scheduled respite session is in August, after which we very much fear that sessions will once again cease as the workers only provide services to children and Christopher is now eighteen years of age.

I have written to the Social Worker, Director of Social Services and to the Chief Executive of the Council regarding our continued difficulties in securing and maintaining a consistent level of respite provision. I have also enquired if respite workers are being sought, or have been located so that sessions will continue, but we have been met with a wall of silence. Sessions remain conditional and have been cancelled or lost through worker absences and the inability to manage mild behaviours. In addition, we have also lost 6 sessions when the respite worker was unable to locate the caretaker of the hall, who retains the key.

Christopher has only one year remaining at school but no transitional planning has been achieved and no day-care placement has been located. At his last ever annual school review held on 14 June 2006 we learned that the adult social worker, who had been introduced to us some weeks earlier, had been replaced by the senior practitioner. Through no fault of her own she had only been passed Christopher's file on the eve of the review and was unable to make a positive contribution to the meeting, despite the situation now being at crisis point.

In 2002 we first contacted our local AM and four years later she is still involved with our case. We are also in contact with the Minister of Health and Social Services, the Councillor of Social Services, The Local Government Ombudsman and of course, our own Solicitor. We continue to write to the Council Solicitor and the Social Services Department to attempt to resolve the situation, but our letters are typically ignored.

We do not know what the future holds for our family and as one battle ends, so another begins. The only thing that has ever remained unchanged throughout the years is our love for our son and our determination to do right by him, and for him, regardless of the opposition.

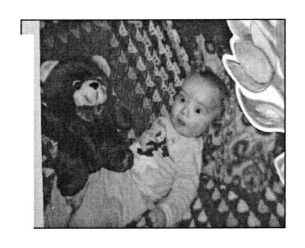

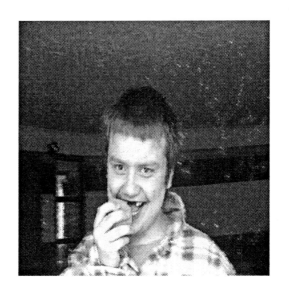

Printed in the United Kingdom
by Lightning Source UK Ltd.
118082UK00001B/151-159